HERBAL MEDICINE FOR MENTAL HEALTH

HERBAL MEDICINE FOR MENTAL HEALTH

Natural Remedies for Anxiety, Depression, ADHD, and More

•••••••••••••••••••••

DR. LILLIAN SOMNER

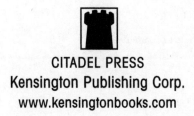

CITADEL PRESS
Kensington Publishing Corp.
www.kensingtonbooks.com

CITADEL PRESS BOOKS are published by

Kensington Publishing Corp. 119
West 40th Street
New York, NY 10018

PUBLISHER'S NOTE
This book is sold to readers with the understanding that while the publisher aims to inform, enlighten, and provide accurate general information regarding the subject matter covered, the publisher is not engaged in providing medical, psychological, financial, legal, or other professional services. If the reader needs or wants professional advice or assistance, the services of an appropriate professional should be sought. Case studies featured in this book are composites based on the author's years of practice and do not reflect the experiences of any individual person.

All Kensington titles, imprints, and distributed lines are available at special quantity discounts for bulk purchases for sales promotions, premiums, fund-raising, educational, or institutional use. Special book excerpts or customized printings can also be created to fit specific needs. For details, write or phone the office of the Kensington sales manager: Kensington Publishing Corp., 119 West 40th Street, New York, NY 10018, attn: Sales Department; phone 1-800-221-2647.

CITADEL PRESS and the Citadel logo are Reg. U.S. Pat. & TM Off.

ISBN: 978-0-8065-4110-5

First Citadel trade paperback printing: April 2022

10 9 8 7 6 5 4 3 2 1

Printed in the United States of America

Electronic edition:

ISBN: 978-0-8065-4111-2 (e-book)

*This book is dedicated
to all who aspire to use the wisdom and history
of the original traditional medicine,
medicine from the plants.*

The doctor of the future will give no medicine
but will instruct his patient in the care of the human frame,
in diet, and in the cause and prevention of disease.

—THOMAS EDISON

CONTENTS

FOREWORD
By Daniel G. Amen, MD

At Amen Clinics, our patients often ask us about medications versus natural solutions for psychiatric, cognitive, and behavioral issues. As a general rule, our psychiatrists, integrative/functional medicine physicians, naturopathic doctors, and other specialists are not opposed to prescription medications . . . *when they are necessary*. However, we firmly believe that pharmaceutical medications should never be the first and only thing you do to help your brain and your mind.

I first became interested in using natural solutions for mental health issues after I started using brain SPECT imaging over thirty years ago. SPECT (single photon emission computed tomography) is an imaging tool that measures blood flow and activity in the brain. It reveals areas with healthy activity, too little activity, and too much activity. On the scans, I could see that some of the psychiatric medications typically prescribed, especially benzodiazepines for anxiety and opiates for pain, were clearly associated with brains that looked unhealthy.

Prescription medications are also linked to a host of unwanted side effects. For example, antidepressants are associated with weight gain, and sexual dysfunction and anti-anxiety pills can make people feel fatigued and bring on brain fog. In additon, with some medications, once you start taking them, you may have a hard time stopping. Withdrawing from antidepressant or anti-anxiety medication can be very difficult.

This inspired me to look for the least toxic, most effective treatments that are supported by scientific studies. It dramatically changed the way we treat our patients. After nearly forty years as a psychiatrist, I recommend more and more treatments from nature, including foods and nutraceuticals.

Many of our patients are equally interested in herbal medicine. This time-honored practice of using plants as medicine to treat disease also includes the treatment of mental health issues. At Amen Clinics, we are fortunate to have on our team Dr. Lillian Somner, a psychiatrist and osteopathic physician who is also trained in herbal medicine. When patients or other physicians inquire about herbal medicine options, I often consult with Dr. Somner.

Now I can point people to her book, *Herbal Medicine for Mental Health*. This valuable resource explores the fascinating history of the ancient practice of herbal medicine along with the wealth of modern-day science supporting it. In an engaging writing style, this book answers so many of the questions I hear from patients and from other psychiatrists, including how herbal medicine compares to functional medicine and homeopathic medicine, how safe it is, as well as how it can be used to treat mental health issues such as depression, anxiety, bipolar disorder, sleep issues, and chronic pain. A series of intriguing case studies from Dr. Somner's real-life patients at Amen Clinics helps bring this book alive.

I think of *Herbal Medicine for Mental Health* as a must-read reference book for every psychiatrist and functional medicine doctor, as well as other physicians who want to expand their knowledge about natural treatments. And for anyone who is struggling with mental health issues and looking for solutions beyond conventional pharmaceuticals, it is an ideal introduction to the world of herbal medicine and the powerful impact it can have in changing people's lives for the better.

INTRODUCTION

I never even used to look at the introduction to books, but now I read them all the time. I do so because it gives me some insight into the author; I can understand their point of view, what has influenced them, and *how* they think. Then I read the book to find out *what* they think.

So, let me give you a window into who I am and how I think. I would like to share my journey into the integration of herbal medicine into my practice as a psychiatrist.

After I graduated from medical school, I was interested in learning about herbs because I wanted to use herbs instead of medication in the treatment of my patients. Of course, it meant learning a whole new world of medicine. I had just finished my studies and I was tired. I decided to put my interest in the botanical world to the side and earn a living to pay back my medical school loans. Twenty years later I came back full circle.

I love what I do. I have been a psychiatrist for more than two decades. But I have not only been a psychiatrist. I am an osteopathic physician and utilized manual therapy in a pain management practice for many years, including many years during which I also practiced as a psychiatrist, with the two interests overlapping. The hands-on work develops a level of understanding and intimacy with patients; it connects the humanity of the practitioner with the humanity of the patient. My osteopathic training instilled in me the understanding that man is triune: body, mind, and spirit. Every osteopathic conference I attended began with this premise. The other osteopathic principles are that the body is a self-regulating, self-healing mechanism, that the body is a whole and that structure and function are related. These are timeless truths. Removing the barriers to health and function is the job of the doctor.

I am also trained in medical acupuncture, a sophisticated application of Chinese energetic medicine to Western medical practice. It is through acupuncture that I first was exposed to the idea that the patient has specific, characteristic ways of manifesting behavior and pathology based on their underlying biopsychotype. In acupuncture assessment there are six structural biopsychotypes that describe a person's normal constitution and characteristic presentations that may lead to pathological presentations common to that type. The biopsychotypes are believed to be the result of the relationship between the energetics of the underlying organs and their related meridians. Identifying the biopsychotype of a given patient is critical for a proper assessment of the pathology they present and how to develop a treatment plan. This is very different from the one-size-fits-all approach of allopathic medicine.

Armed with these ideas, I treated patients in a private psychiatric practice for many years. The conventional diagnostic approach (using the DSM, *Diagnostic Statistical Manual*, the psychiatrist's standard of care) was limited and did not seem to capture a good understanding of the patient in front of me. I did not get good results from prescribing medication; there were many failures of treatment and many untoward side effects. Let me pause here to stress that medication can be very important and helpful, and there were some patients who I successfully treated using just pharmaceuticals. I studied functional medicine through the A4M (American Academy of Anti-aging Medicine) and also through the Institute for Functional Medicine, and began expanding my treatment options into exercise, nutrition, and dietary supplements. The dietary supplements were mostly amino acids with a smattering of herbs. Lifestyle medicine became the foundation of my work. Therapy and the processing of emotions were also central. This is very difficult to accomplish since it takes a long time and is painful work. We live in a world of instant gratification and a pill for everything, so therapy is not the top treatment of choice for most patients, although it is very effective.

Then in 2009, I met Dr. Daniel Amen and learned about using SPECT (single proton emission computerized tomography) scans as a diagnostic tool. Dr. Amen has developed protocols for the management of specific SPECT scan findings that are very helpful. The scans give a direct picture into the specific organ associated with psychological processes: the brain. The brain is responsible for interpreting our life events and making decisions about them. Understanding the brain and utilizing the brain scans help us to create a treatment plan that will make a difference to the patient in a deep and meaningful way.

All of this is helpful for determining a diagnosis and developing a treatment plan. I still found that the use of supplements was not sufficient to make the shift in patient care that I wanted to see. My good friend and colleague, Inga Wieser, was making big shifts in patients in her private practice as a master herbalist and aromatherapist. She re-ignited my fire regarding herbal medicine, and I took the Foundations in Herbal Medicine course with Dr. Tieraona Low Dog and was hooked. Dr. Low Dog's way of teaching is practical, and I implemented what I learned from her immediately into clinical practice, and soon my patients were getting better results with fewer side effects. When I treat a patient, I use everything: medication, functional medicine, lifestyle medicine, SPECT scans and the appropriate protocols, and of course, the herbs. I have also since completed a certification fellowship in herbal medicine offered by the American Academy of Restorative Medicine.

As a perpetual student, I did my research. I looked for a book that was written by a psychiatrist for psychiatrists to show me the path of how to use these great herbs I was learning about. There are none. I looked for books that explain the use of herbs for psychological issues in general and could find none. What I did find were websites, some more helpful than others, but none by licensed professionals. There are self-help books, but none that focused specifically on herbs, making their use front and center of the treatment plan.

I think one reason for a lack of books that explain the use of herbs for psychological issues is that, like medical acupuncture, herbal medicine views psychological issues as simply a part of the whole person, with their specific characteristics and nuances. It is not seen as a pathology on its own. There is no bipolar person in the field of herbal medicine, but rather a particular energetic type that happens to cycle between mania and depressive episodes. What is more important is the specific, underlying energetic type rather than that they happen to cycle. According to herbal medicine, if you treat the underlying energetic distortions along with the cycling you will have more success.

This book is the first foray into bridging the gap between the psychological disorder as the focus and the whole person with a psychological complaint, requiring an individualized treatment approach utilizing herbal medicines as the primary medical approach, along with lifestyle and functional medical treatments. I want this book to make herbal medicine readily available to anyone who wants to try it. Welcome to my journey.

PART I

HERBAL MEDICINE BASICS

1

WHAT IS AN HERB?

In a book concerned with herbal medicine I thought it a good idea to ask, "What exactly is an herb?" What I find fascinating is that none of the herbal medicine textbooks that I have define an herb. As I did more research to find an answer, I came to realize that the definition of an herb has to do with what the person who is defining it is going to do with the herb. For example, an herb is a food if you are going to cook it, eat it, or flavor with it. I consulted my *Chef's Guide*[1] which defines an herb as "leaves of an aromatic plant, usually from a temperate climate." (In case you're curious, a spice is defined as, "Seeds, bark, root, flower, bud, resin, or any other part of an aromatic plant, usually from a tropical climate.") What I find interesting is the need for the plant to be aromatic. Plants with scents are high in volatile oils and many provide essential oils that are used in aromatherapy.

Definition of an Herb

The American Herbalist Guild is the premier organization for not only training people in herbal medicine but promoting the practice in the United States. They define an herb in the context of medicine itself, "Medicinally, an herb is any plant or plant part used for its therapeutic value."

What is clear is that herbs are from a plant, whether they are eaten as food, drunk as a beverage, used as flavoring, or used as a medicine. The various parts of the plant are used in a multitude of ways. For some plants only the roots offer value, while others hold their gifts in their leaves and flowers.

What Exactly Is Herbal Medicine?

We can define herbal medicine (also referred to as phytotherapy) intuitively, just from the words. We now have an understanding of what an herb is and we all have an understanding of medicine as something used to treat illness or disease. Therefore, herbal medicine is the use of herbs as medicine to treat disease. Herbal medicine also includes a concept that is not present in pharmaceutical medicine: tonics. A tonic, or alterative as they are now called, are herbal compounds that nourish and support the health of the system. A further exploration of tonics will be found in later chapters.

Herbal medicine is a time-honored tradition. All peoples have turned to plants for their ailments, no matter where in the world they lived. In ancient times, phytotherapy was all there was. There were only the plants that the local doctor—a shaman or medicine man/woman—knew about and used to treat various conditions. And think about the plants that your mother or grandmother would give you, like chamomile or fennel tea for upset stomach. Herbal medicine is older than Western medicine, which has only existed for a little over five hundred years. Plants have been utilized in the treatment of human and animal ailments for thousands of years. The tradition of medicine was passed down from teacher to student because there was no written word at the time. Indigenous peoples have always used their environment for shelter, clothing, and sustenance. And yes, for medicine.

Most medical practices in the Western world today are based on the medicine of the Greeks, most notably represented by Hippocrates. Hippocrates is credited as the first physician to think that physical disease had a natural cause (rather than the then widely held belief that illness was from a supernatural cause, such as an "arrow" shot from the bow of the Greek god Apollo) and the first to treat it using natural remedies found in nature; that is, the plants. Hippocrates was also the first physician to keep a written record of the treatments he used for his patients. And he also incorporated what we today call lifestyle medicine in his treatment plans— things like exercise, diet, and fresh air. By removing medical treatment from the priests, he opened the door to scientific study of the plants. What is key though, is that he believed that it was not just medicine, but also lifestyle that are needed to bring about health. I will be discussing lifestyle throughout this book.

Is herbal medicine different from allopathic medicine, functional medicine, and homeopathic medicine?

Herbal medicine, as we have seen, is the use of plants as the primary source of treatment for an ailment. It is a full body of medicine and is ancient in its history. By comparison, allopathic medicine is the term used to describe Western medicine. Allopathic medicine is, by and large, using remedies that are the opposite of the symptoms of the disease. For example, a doctor will prescribe a medication to bring down a fever or suppress a cough. The tools of allopathic medicine are pharmaceutical medications along with surgery. The pharmaceutical medications are largely synthetically made in a laboratory.

Functional medicine, a recent development in the practice of medicine, focuses on improving health of the body by optimizing its biological and psychological function. Functional medicine is comprehensive, using the tools of pharmaceutical medicine and herbal medicine. Functional medicine always includes the use of lifestyle medicine as its foundational base.

Homeopathic medicine was developed by Samuel Hahnemann in 1796. The development of homeopathy was in reaction to the practice of medicine at the time. In the 1700s, medicine was practiced utilizing ideas developed by Paracelsus, who is considered to be the father of pharmacology. Paracelsus was an alchemist interested in treating the body with minerals. This is how syphilis came to be treated with mercury (a mineral). The saying, "A night with Venus and a lifetime with mercury" stems from that time and is a reference to the use of mercury for the treatment of syphilis. Hahnemann was disillusioned with the use of mercury due to its toxic effects and began to develop his own ideas and experimentation. Instead of the allopathic treatment principles of opposites, he proposed the treatment of "similars." As stated earlier, in allopathic medicine if you have a fever, you are recommended to take something that will bring the fever down. In homeopathic medicine you will take a highly diluted (so you do not make yourself sick) version of something that would cause the symptoms and *be similar to the whole of who you are*. The American Institute of Homeopathy's website defines homeopathy this way: "The word Homeopathy, which comes from the Greek, through Latin into English, literally means 'like disease.' This means that the medicine given is like the disease that the person is expressing, in his totality, not like a specific disease category or medical diagnosis."

Does herbal medicine utilize essential oils?

Essential oils are the volatile compounds found in a plant. They are volatile in that they are readily released from the plant into the air at normal temperatures and can be smelled easily by someone breathing in their fumes. Essential oils are what give the flower its fragrance. Their uniform characteristic is that they are hydrophobic (water hating) and lipophilic (oil loving). Therefore, the essential oils are more readily blended in oil. They are not oils, themselves, but a wide variety of compounds that are soluble in many different carriers, just not in water. It is because of their aroma that essential oils are used widely in the perfume industry, and it is because of their aroma that essential oil therapy is called aromatherapy. With the advent of essential oil multilevel marketing businesses, the use of essential oils has become more widespread and interest in their medicinal value has grown. Aromatherapy and herbal medicine are two different practices, but they work well together and I use both modalities in my treatment plans.

Herbal Affinity for Specific Organ Systems

There is a concept in herbal medicine that is not present in allopathic medicine. That is the concept of herbal affinity. In medical school I was never taught, "use amoxicillin because it has an affinity for the throat." We do not think like that in allopathic medicine. We think in terms of pharmaceuticals and how they affect the illness or disease. We think, if there is infection, calm it with an anti-infectious agent. Most often the pharmaceutical is designed to slow, reduce, or stop a metabolic process. There are also some medications that are designed to stimulate a process. For example, marinol is used to stimulate the appetite or amphetamine to stimulate the brain.

In herbal medicine, the herbs have wide applications and actions but will have a specific affinity for an organ system. For example, kava kava, well known as an anti-anxiety herb, was brought to the United States initially because of its affinity for the urinary system as a bladder anti-spasmodic. It is known to relax the body but leave the mind alert. Hawthorn has an affinity for the cardiovascular system. Raspberry leaf has an affinity for the uterus. In herbal medicine, an herb is used not only for the action needed, but for its affinity for the organ in question. For example, chamomile has anti-spasmodic effects. It also has an affinity for the gastrointestinal system. So, if you have cramping in the intestine, you would choose chamomile because of its affinity for the gastrointestinal system as well as its anti-spasmodic effects. If you have a muscle spasm in your calf you would choose the anti-spasmodic cramp bark because of its affinity for muscle cramps.

Herbs often have multiple actions and an affinity for

multiple parts of the body. Black cohosh, for example, has anti-inflammatory actions and pain-relieving actions for the joints and muscles of the body. It was historically used as a remedy for rheumatic pain in the joints, such as osteoarthritis. However, it is also helpful for treating the deep, dark moods, referred to as melancholy, that descend on people. These moods may be episodic, sometimes coming with the menstrual cycle, and can be quite dark.

Some herbal actions are expected based on the plant's appearance or natural function. Black cohosh has light, beautiful racemes on the top of the plant with deep, dark, tangled roots underneath. It is a tangled mess on the inside (the roots) and beautiful on the outside. So, we would expect the plant to work with a person who feels all knotted up on the inside but is put together on the outside. Pleurisy root is a plant that resembles the lungs. Pleurisy root has a strong affinity for the lung and the pleura (a thin membrane that covers the inside surface of the rib cage and spreads over the lungs as well) in particular. Comfrey grows wildly and in just about any environment. It is known as a regenerator of tissue. Dr. Tieraona Low Dog shared a personal experience of using comfrey to treat the bed sore of a dying man. The man had little vitality since he was dying, but the comfrey was able to begin the repair process of that deep wound within twenty-four hours.

In pharmaceutical medicine there is an attempt to isolate the one chemical, the one action for which that medication is indicated. In herbal medicine the same herb may be used for a variety of symptoms. Black cohosh, mentioned above, is also used in the treatment of asthma or bronchitis. To the pharmaceutically oriented physician it seems peculiar to use the same remedy for asthma and joint pain. In herbal medicine this is commonplace. Herbs are often prescribed together because their synergistic action is more potent than their action as a single compound. For example, black cohosh is often used with the herb lobelia for asthma.

The hunt for the one compound in an herb that provides the benefit is ongoing in scientific studies. Sometimes the one compound *is* identified, isolated, and synthesized, and used for medication. For example, curcumin is the anti-inflammatory compound found in turmeric root.

Is Herbal Medicine Safe?

While I was writing this book, my husband asked me how I was going to explain the use of the herbs when there was no scientific study on them. This is a common misconception in herbal medicine, but the truth is that many of the herbs are well studied. Sure, not *all* herbs have been scientifically studied, but not all herbs need to be studied. If we know the constituents of the herb and know what those constituents do, we will know what the herb does. It is not necessary to test each herb individually.

One question on everyone's mind regarding herbal medicine is safety. In the United States we are accustomed to being told a drug is safe based on scientific testing and passing rigorous demands placed by the Food and Drug Administration (FDA). Consequently, we take our medications with a sense of comfort knowing that the medications being prescribed to us by the medical field are scientifically tested. Faced with an herb, something that is not tested by the FDA, that feeling of safety and confidence is lacking. It is completely appropriate to wonder if something you are going to take or give to your family is safe.

How do we know if an herbal preparation is safe? Or effective? In herbal medicine the answer is twofold: it is in time-honored tradition and in scientific study. Both have happened. There are many scientific studies done on plants and herbs.

In time-honored tradition, the same, or similar herb can be found around the world. That same herb has been used by indigenous cultures for the same thing for centuries. Time-honored tradition across cultures is one way we know how to use an herb. It is also how we know what is poisonous and what should not be eaten.

Turmeric is an example of a time-honored herb used for centuries in Ayurvedic medicine. Turmeric is a member of the *Zingirberaceae* family, from which we get ginger. Turmeric also shares many of the same benefits as ginger. In ancient times, turmeric was given for the treatment of inflammation of the gastrointestinal tract, to improve gastritis, and for use in relieving pain and inflammation in the body. If turmeric was to be used for reducing inflammation in the gastrointestinal tract it was given mixed in food without fat or pepper or taken on an empty stomach. If it was to be given as an aid for inflammation in the rest of the body it was made into a food with fat, usually ghee, and pepper.

The current scientific research on turmeric shows that the active constituent of turmeric is curcumin. There are numerous research articles written on the study of curcumin. A current PubMed request yielded 14,557 articles. *Alternative Medicine Review* (Volume 14, Number 2, 2009) has an excellent article demonstrating the vast research done on curcumin. It has been shown to heal ulcers in the stomach, improve colorectal cancer, reduce the risk of cancer of a variety of types (due to its anti-inflammatory effects), improve ulcerative colitis, and when given as a preparation that is absorbable, it is helpful for osteoarthritis and rheumatoid arthritis. Curcumin is not well absorbed from the gastrointestinal tract. It is also rapidly cleared from the serum. Studies have shown that curcumin's absorption through the intestinal tract is enabled with the aid of pepper, more specifically the alkaloid, piperine. The addition of piperine increased the absorption twenty-fold. There you have it: time-honored tradition proven by science.

There has been a lot of scientific research done on plants to identify their biochemical constituents. We do not need placebo controlled, double blind studies on each herb when the actions of the constituents are well known. For example, marshmallow root (*Althaea officinalis*) and slippery elm bark (*Ulmus rubra*) are used for similar ailments because both of them are mucilaginous demulcents. A mucilaginous plant is one that swells when exposed to water and creates a mucilage (mucus like) film that soothes and protects tissues. These two herbs are used regularly for the treatment of gastritis, reflux, and cough. Any time mucosal tissue needs soothing, both of these plants will be effective. Knowing their constituents (the mucilage) will allow you to know how the plant will behave and thus, specific studies on each plant may not be necessary.

A note about how herbal medicine is made. As consumers we are accustomed to going to a pharmacy and picking up a prescription ordered for us by our physician. Most of the time this pharmaceutical comes in the form of a pill. We are also familiar with some medications as a liquid, such as a cough medicine. We are also familiar with injections.

Herbal medicine is different. The herbal remedies often come in the form of a tincture or an extract. This is made by subjecting the herb to a solvent to extract constituents out of the plant. The most common solvent is alcohol, but other solvents may be used as well. Because I recommend the use of the herbal preparations over a prolonged period of time, I have a personal preference for alcohol-free extracts called glycerites. These extracts are made using glycerin and water as the solvent.

The remedy may also be in the form of dried or fresh herb (the parts of the plant that are above ground known as aerial parts), or dried or fresh roots. The herb and/or roots may also be made into a tea to drink. The most common teas are made from the aerial parts and simply steeped in water, water being the solvent. A decoction is defined as simmering the herb, steeping the herbs, and then drinking the resultant tea. Decoctions are usually used to pull the constituents out of roots or thick, woody stems.

2

DIAGNOSIS

The diagnosis is how a doctor makes sense of the symptoms and complaints the patient presents. The diagnosis is what allows the doctor to figure out what treatment or treatments will help the patient feel better. Having an accurate diagnosis is imperative for the success of the treatment. However, an accurate diagnosis is not always easy, and the disorder may change and evolve. Therefore, the diagnosis may change and evolve as well.

How a diagnosis is made depends on which type of medicine you are practicing. Western allopathic medicine, Chinese medicine, and Western herbal medicine all have completely different foci, and treatment approaches can also vary. What distinguishes the Eastern traditional diagnosis process is the concept of life force (also referred to as energy or Qi). The Eastern practitioner utilizes the energetic imbalances for their diagnosis. In Western allopathic medicine, we make the diagnosis based on symptoms, physical exam, laboratory tests, and images. The Western herbal approach is more similar to the Western allopathic approach, but also recognizes the nuances of the individual. In allopathic medicine, the disease state is the main focus, but in Western herbal medicine, the person as a whole is the main focus. Herbal medicine looks at the person who has the disorder, rather than what disorder the patient has.

Let's look at how depression is diagnosed by each approach.

Allopathic medical diagnosis for a major depressive episode is based on a constellation of symptoms experienced over a period of time. According to the DSM (the *Diagnostic and Statistical Manual*, the diagnostic manual for psychiatrists) one must have five or more of the following symptoms over a two-week period:

- Depressed mood, more days than not
- Markedly diminished pleasure in all or most activities, nearly every day
- Significant change in weight or appetite; either weight gain or weight loss
- A slowing down of thought and a reduction of physical movement noticeable to others (cannot be just personal self-perception)
- Fatigue or loss of energy nearly every day
- Feelings of worthlessness or feelings of inappropriate guilt, nearly every day
- Diminished ability to think or concentrate, or indecisiveness, nearly every day
- Recurrent thoughts of death, recurrent suicidal ideation without a specific plan, or a suicide attempt or a specific suicide plan

These symptoms must interfere with the person's life and not be the result of another illness or of substance abuse.

The diagnosis of major depressive episode is made by interview, known as the mental status exam. The mental status exam is a combination of asking questions of the patient (e.g., asking how they feel) and the doctor's observations of the patient, called objective signs. The doctor will want to rule out any physical causes of the mood and will order blood work to make sure there is no underlying medical cause of the depressed mood.

An integrative medicine physician would also perform a mental status exam but would be more comprehensive in the blood work. The integrative physician may look for signs of inflammation and infection as well as hormonal imbalance, all of which can contribute to mood disorders.

Dr. Daniel Amen is the first to add imaging studies to the diagnosis of psychiatric disorders. Below are two SPECT scan

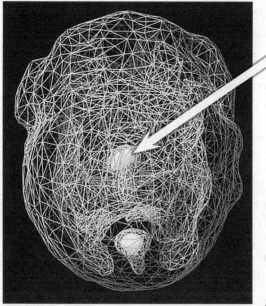

Note the overactive limbic system

Fig 2.1 Image of a brain showing depressive disorder. *Used with patient permission.*

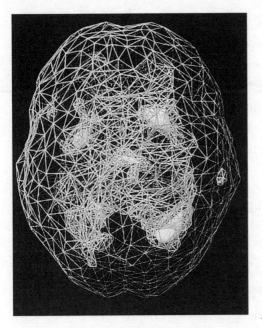

Fig 2.2 Scan of a brain with normal activity. *Amen Clinic Library. Used with permission.*

images of the brain. Figure 2.1 is an image of a brain with depressed disorder. The limbic system is overly active and associated with depressed mood.

Notice the difference in the scan of a brain with normal activity (Figure 2.2).

Chinese energetic medicine has a completely different method of diagnosis. I trained in Acupuncture Energetics with Dr. Joseph Helms. Dr. Helms teaches medical acupuncture to physicians and medically trained personnel only through the Helms Medical Institute in Berkeley, California, the oldest and best-known acupuncture training program for physicians. This system is different from the Traditional Chinese Medicine system (TCM) that is more familiar to the public. The acupuncture system of TCM is based on the herbal model rather than the energetic model. What I will discuss here, however, is the energetic model. Please note that the discussion here is very brief and does not represent the full medical system that forms Chinese energetic medicine.

According to energetic medicine, there are six basic energies and twelve meridians derived from them. Each meridian system is related to an energetic organ system with functional influence. Here are the twelve meridians:

- Lung meridian
- Pericardium meridian
- Heart meridian
- Colon meridian
- Triple warmer meridian
- Intestinal meridian
- Urinary bladder meridian
- Stomach meridian
- Liver meridian
- Spleen meridian
- Kidney meridian
- Gall bladder meridian

The diagnostic assessment of the patient utilizing these principles categorizes symptoms according to the meridian/organ system that is perturbed and establishes the energetic equation. How one determines the energetic equation is to place the primary complaints in a particular energetic axis and then establish which axis is primary, which axis is secondary, and which axis is constitutional. The treatment intervention is determined by the complaint that is the most problematic for the patient. That complaint will be treated first, but the practitioner will address each axis at every visit. The energetic equation is re-evaluated at each visit and adjustments to the treatment approach may be made.

So, a patient presenting with depressive feelings may be diagnosed as suffering from depression, but those feelings are only one part of their energetic equation. And the depressive feelings may be addressed immediately since it is the reason the patient came to the doctor, but all of the energetic axes will be included in the treatment plan.

Western herbal medicine is different from all of the above. It does not utilize the energetic equation directly, but the energetics of the herb may come into play. By that I mean it considers whether an herb is cooling or warming, or has a particular characteristic that is important because it resonates with the characteristic of the patient. The patient is assessed in a way similar to the allopathic evaluation with medical history and physical exam, but herbal medicine also takes into account the characteristic of the patient and how it relates to the characteristics of the herb that will be used to treat the patient. For example, David Winston, a well-known herbalist and sought-after teacher and speaker, defines thirteen different types of depression. Each one is dependent on the overall context of the person's life, and the herbalist seeks to find an underlying root cause for the depression. (We will explore the different types of depression in the next section of this book.) For example, a common type of depression is the GI depression. An important aspect of the history taking for anyone who has the complaint of depression is to assess the state of the digestive system. Is there reflux? Bloating after a meal? Has there been a diagnosis of irritable bowel syndrome? The answers to these and other questions direct the treatment. Evidence shows there is a relationship between the gut and the brain, and those with inflammation have a much higher risk of developing depressed mood.

So, if indicated, an herbal treatment for gut inflammation would be prescribed.

In Western herbal medicine there are also herbal treatments for depression related to hormone imbalance, unrelieved grief, and nutrient deficiencies. The herbal treatments are designed to improve the mood, but also to treat the underlying imbalance and give herbal remedies that support the underlying issues.

The diagnostic method used in herbal medicine demonstrates an interest in the whole person and the details regarding the symptoms of depressed mood. It is the understanding of the person, their traits, and their underlying constitution that are of prime importance. The focus is on the patient as a whole, rather than the disease state.

PART II

HERBAL MEDICINE FOR DEPRESSION

3

DEPRESSION

Major depression is one of the most common and devastating mental health disorders in the United States. It is a disabling condition that brings untoward suffering to the person who has the condition and to those who love them. According to the National Institute of Mental Health, an organization that tracks prevalence of mental health disorders, approximately 7 percent of all U.S. adults (defined as 18 years of age and older) have had an episode of depression, with the highest prevalence in the 18- to 25-year age range. (Note, however, the most recent data on their website as of this writing is from 2017.) Those reporting to be biracial (any two races) had the highest incidence of depressive episodes. Women were more likely to experience depression than men, and 64 percent of adults with the disorder experienced severe impairment. The prevalence of depression in adolescents (defined as age 12–17) is 13.3 percent. This translates to approximately 3.2 million adolescents. Again, the prevalence is higher in girls than boys. Adolescents reporting to be biracial (any two races) had the highest incidence of depressive episodes. Seventy percent of adolescents with the disorder experienced severe impairment.

These are disturbing statistics.

As stated in the previous chapter, according to the DSM-5, a diagnosis of depression is based on having five or more of the following symptoms over a two-week period:

- Depressed mood, more days than not
- Markedly diminished pleasure in all or most activities, nearly every day
- Significant change in weight or appetite; either weight gain or weight loss
- A slowing down of thought and a reduction of physical movement noticeable to others (cannot be just personal self-perception)
- Fatigue or loss of energy nearly every day
- Feelings of worthlessness or feelings of inappropriate guilt, nearly every day
- Diminished ability to think or concentrate, or indecisiveness, nearly every day
- Recurrent thoughts of death, recurrent suicidal ideation without a specific plan, or a suicide attempt or a specific suicide plan

These symptoms must interfere with life and not be due to a medical condition or substance abuse.

Types of Depression

Certainly, depression is the most common mental health diagnosis that I address in my practice. There are many different types of depression recognized by the psychiatric field. Postpartum depression is the most common negative consequence of pregnancy. Psychotic depression is a severe form of depression during which the individual loses touch with reality. Bipolar depression—deep depressive episodes following periods of mania (high energy often accompanied by poor judgment)—can be very deep and difficult to diagnose. Treatment-resistant depression is a type of depression that has not responded to treatment and is persistent and disabling. There is cyclic depression called cyclothymia, seasonal affective depression, and depressed mood that comes with premenstrual syndrome.

Hormonal issues, such as an imbalance of hormones or thyroid issues, may underlie the depressed mood. One can also have depression because they are completely burned out from stress, and the hormonal system, the hypothalamic pituitary adrenal (HPA) axis, is no longer able to manage the chronic stress level. When stress is chronic and cortisol, the stress hormone, is chronically high, it can cause a melancholic depression. Someone who is burned out from stress and whose adrenal gland is not able to make an adequate amount of cortisol to support the psyche of the person can also experience depression. This is an atypical depression.

Head injury may also damage the brain and contribute to depression, anxiety, and insomnia. At the Amen clinic, we see brain injury as a common occurrence with psychiatric disorders.

Sometimes a depression comes as the result of a life experience, such as a great loss, known as adjustment disorder with depressed mood. There is also dysthymia, a persistent feeling of blah, a depressed state that persisted for two years or more but does not meet the criteria for major depression. Suicidal thoughts are not a type of depression, but a state of mind associated with depressed mood, specifically hopelessness.

In herbal medicine there are other types of depression. Depression may be related to the liver, with anger as a primary symptom. Depression may be related to the inability to process loss or being stuck. It may be related to inflammation in the gastrointestinal tract causing inflammation in the brain via the gut-brain connection.

Diagnostic and Treatment Differences Between Allopathic Medicine and Herbal Medicine

When looking at a person who feels depressed through the lens of herbal medicine, there are many questions to ask before determining a treatment plan. Let's look at an example of a patient I evaluated.

Amelia is a thirty-eight-year-old woman who came to the clinic complaining of being overwhelmed by her life. She complains of feelings of depressed mood that come and go, accompanied by feelings of hopelessness. These feelings have been present for years. She has been hospitalized for suicide attempts three times in the past. When she feels overwhelmed, she gets angry and depressed, and these feelings worsen with her menstrual cycle. She has digestive distress and is an emotional overeater although she works as a dietician for a diabetic clinic and has an interest in nutrition. She complains of difficulty with focus, a lifelong struggle but now it is interfering with her work.

She is raising three children on her own; their father is a drug addict and in and out of jail. She still loves him, but she is on her own most of the time. She lost the women leaders in her life; her mother and both grandmothers died within a short time of one another. Since the loss of her mother, her disabled brother has become another burden for her.

Amelia drinks more than she thinks she should, drinking wine or vodka seltzers more days a week than not. She has trouble falling asleep and waking up, so she is chronically tired with little energy.

Take a moment to think about this history. Is it one you can relate to? How do you respond when you feel overwhelmed and your life is out of control? How do you respond when you have more responsibility than you can manage?

Amelia's case is fairly complicated but is common in our clinic. Her case presents many of the types of depression that are listed above and will be discussed at length below.

She meets criteria for dysthymia, the type of depression that is less severe than the major depressive disorder but is long standing (greater than two years) punctuated by episodes of major depression. A conventional psychiatrist would appropriately refer her for cognitive behavioral therapy and offer an anti-depressant medication. If the conventional psychiatrist was thorough, Amelia might also receive a blood test for TSH (thyroid stimulating hormone), vitamin B12, and vitamin D. However, if that is all that is done for Amelia there is a lot missing.

If she saw a psychiatrist trained in herbal medicine, she would receive a more comprehensive blood workup to include more aspects of the thyroid function including a test for antibodies to the thyroid hormone. Along with the measurement of her vitamin D level, some key minerals (copper, zinc, and ferritin) including the intracellular level of magnesium would be measured. Magnesium has a large influence on anxiety and tension. Perhaps most importantly, she would have the stress hormone cortisol measured. We need to see if she is still very high on the stress level or if she has burned out and dropped low. Diet, exercise, and stress management would all be included in the evaluation. A psychiatrist trained in herbal medicine would address her specific issues influenced by her symptoms in all areas of her life, not just her mood.

The way I understand her is that she has moods that cycle throughout the week and with her menstrual cycle, so there is a hormonal component to her moodiness. She has difficulty with her digestion, so there is a gastrointestinal component to her depression. She complained of feelings of being overwhelmed, which is another word for anxiety and burnout. She complained about focus difficulties (the SPECT scans we took at the Amen Clinic confirm attention deficits are likely). Difficulties in sleep and difficulties waking up were also issues. The difficulty in waking up can be related to a low cortisol level, and she could be in the burnout phase of her stress pattern. She has a "liver" component because of the anger she experiences along with the depressed mood. If she is just given the recommendation of therapy (which I think she needs) and/or an anti-depressant medication the doctor would be missing these underlying con-tributing factors.

The herbal medicine approach is to look at the herbal actions that are needed.

Herbal Actions Needed and Common Herbs with Those Actions

Anti-depressants	Lemon balm
	Black cohosh
	Vitex
	Bupleurum
	Turmeric
	Night blooming cereus
Anti-anxiety	Passionflower
	Motherwort
	Tiger lily
	Kava kava
	Bacopa monnieri
	California poppy
	Hops
	Valerian
	Milky oats
Nervous system alternatives (tonics) For nourishment of the nervous system	Bacopa monnieri
	St. John's wort
	Milky oats
	Skullcap
	Passionflower
	Valerian
	Chamomile
	Lemon balm

Adaptogens to support the overall stress level	Licorice
	Ashwagandha
	Eleuthero
	Schisandra
	Rhodiola
	Ginseng
	Holy basil
Bitters to help her digestive complaints	Hops
	Motherwort
	Blue vervain
	Artichoke
	Dandelion root

For the hormonal component, I recommended *Vitex agnus-castus* (chasteberry) and black cohosh (*Actaea racemosa*) to improve and level her mood. The chasteberry will increase the progesterone at the last portion of the cycle, which will lessen her premenstrual symptoms. Black cohosh is used for the dark moods that are cyclic in nature. I recommended to her Nature's Way 540 mg capsule of black cohosh, taken once daily.

For the angry component, I recommended bupleurum, an excellent tonic for the liver, a bitter herb that clears heat from the liver. In Chinese medicine, the liver is where anger is felt and when it gets hot, it explodes into irritability. Bupleurum is a bitter, which will also improve her digestive symptoms. Bupleurum can be taken as an alcohol-free tincture mixed in water. Hawaii Pharm makes an alcohol-free tincture. I recommended Amelia take 1 ml three times a day.

For the anxiety and difficulty with focus (a lifelong complaint that is interfering with her work), I recommended Bacopa monnieri, which will help improve her focus along with improving the anxiety and worry. Bacopa monnieri is also a nervous system tonic. Himalaya makes a 750 mg caplet to be taken once daily.

For the adaptogen (healing herb that helps with stress and anxiety), I recommended licorice. Licorice is very well researched and how it works is well-known. Cortisol is the hormone that manages stress, and licorice helps the cortisol our body makes stick around longer. Amelia is burned out, as evidenced by her difficulty waking up in the morning and her feelings of being overwhelmed. Improving her cortisol level may be very helpful for her.

A note about licorice: Some practitioners are afraid of using licorice. Licorice contains a compound called glycyrrhizin, which inhibits the excretion of sodium and increases the excretion of potassium in the kidney, raising the blood pressure. It is important to keep the whole licorice dose at 1000 mg or less daily to avoid the blood pressure issue. If the patient has any blood pressure problems, I recommend monitoring the blood pressure and also keeping the dose of whole licorice below 1000 mg daily.

Herbs Used for Depression

Important Note: If you suffer from any type of depression, *please* see a qualified practitioner. The herbs listed below are *not* a substitute for professional medical guidance. They are also not to be all used together. Which ones to use, how and when, are determined by the totality of the person.

The herbal medicine materia medica for the treatment of depression was detailed by David Winston, RH (AHG) in his work entitled *Differential Treatment of Depression and Anxiety with Botanical and Nutritional Medicines,* originally copyrighted 2006 and revised 2016. It is available online and I recommend it as an excellent read for this topic.

The following herbs are a sampling from that original work to give some examples of how to match the herb with the depression type. What you will notice is that unlike pharmaceutical approaches, which focus on the neurotransmitter receptor site and follow only the serotonin or dopamine causes of depression, herbs focus on supporting the underlying metabolic system that is functioning in a suboptimal manner leading to depressed mood. This philosophical difference is the most profound difference between conventional psychiatry and herbal medicine for psychiatric disorders.

Below are the most common herbal recommendations for depression. The different categories of depression are discussed in detail in the following chapters.

GI-Based Depression

St. John's wort (*Hypericum perforatum*) has a well-known reputation as an anti-depressant and may be familiar to the reader. It is considered effective for the treatment of mild to moderate depression. It has many properties and indications beyond depression, including digestive aid, increasing the release of bile, and antiulcer. It is available as a tea, tincture, extract, or pill. Extracts are typically standardized to the hypericin (the chemical thought to be responsible for the benefit) content. The typical dose of St. John's wort is 900–1200 mg in divided doses over the course of the day, standardized to 0.35 hypericin; whole herb capsules are 500–1500 mg, three to four times a day. I have recommended to take it all at bedtime when sleep is difficult. It is very relaxing. St. John's wort is available as an herb at a local herb store or an online herb store such as www.mountainroseherbs.com or www.starwest-botanicals.com. If taken as a tea, it is recommended that you drink 4–8 ounces, one to four times per day. It has a pleasant flavor. St. John's wort will interact with medications so caution should be used if you are taking prescription medicines. Seek the advice of a qualified practitioner. Do *not* take with cyclosporin or birth control pills.

Saffron (*Crocus sativus*). Saffron is best known as a culinary herb in the United States but it has been used as a dye and valued for its aroma in other countries. Maud Grieve, simply known as Mrs. Grieve (a highly regarded herbal historian), in *A Modern Herbal* wrote that saffron originated in Persia and was taken to Spain, which currently supplies most of the saffron we use today. Thomas Easley, herbalist and co-author of *The Modern Herbal Dispensatory*, describes the herb's effect as a potent anti-inflammatory for the "cytokines (chemicals our body makes when inflammation is needed) associated with depression."[2] Saffron also has the properties of being a carminative (an herb that reduces intestinal gas, a mild laxative, and an emetic.)[3] The limiting factor in the use of saffron is its cost. It takes 14,000 saffron threads to produce one ounce of saffron. There are only three saffron threads per flower and no mechanized way of separating them from the plant. So, it is very labor intensive to produce saffron. For this reason, it is very expensive. Luckily only a small amount of it is needed so the cost can be minimized. A well-advertised version of this herb is Satiereal® which has been studied for appetite management. For depression, the dose is 20–30 mg daily of an extract available as a capsule. Dr. Amen has developed two products that contain saffron, Serotonin Mood Support and Happy Saffron. Both are available online at www.brainmd.com.

Evening primrose leaf, root bark, flower, and oil (*Oenothera biennis*). Evening primrose is a beautiful wildflower plant with yellow flowers. The entire plant is edible and if grown in the garden, you can eat the leaves and flowers in a salad and eat the roots prepared as a potato. As the name implies, this plant blooms in the evening. According to David Winston, evening primrose is perfect for the depression associated with significant stomach distress such as indigestion, nausea, and vomiting. The depression is one of apathy and a gloomy mood. Dr. James Duke, in *Handbook of Medicinal Herbs,* presents the indications for evening primrose oil as anxiety, diarrhea, and dyspepsia among many others. It is thought that GLA (the omega 6 gamma linoleic acid) is the primary anti-depressant ingredient in evening primrose oil. Winston recommends taking the tincture, but it is not commercially available. What is commercially available is the evening primrose oil, compressed from the seeds of the plant. Take 1300 mg daily. It is not for use during pregnancy.

Liver Based Depression

St. John's wort (*Hypericum perforatum*). See above.

Rosemary (*Rosmarinus officinalis*). Rosemary will surely be familiar as a culinary herb frequently used in Mediterranean cooking. It is widely available as a fresh herb in the supermarket and can easily be grown in your home garden. Rosemary is known for its ability to combat brain fog, improve cognition and cerebral circulation, and improve mood. It is included under the liver-based depression section because of its beneficial effects as an herb that is hepatoprotective (prevents damage to the liver). It is helpful to treat depression in combination with St. John's wort and evening primrose oil (see above). Rosemary can be taken as a tea and may be mixed with other teas for flavoring. Put one teaspoon of the leaf in a cup of hot water, steep for 5–7 minutes, strain, and drink. The recommended dose is 1–2 cups daily. Rosemary is also available as an extract in capsule form. Nature's Way makes a preparation of 350 mg in 2 capsules to be taken twice daily. The culinary use of rosemary is safe during pregnancy, but the medicinal doses should not be taken during pregnancy, or given to small children.

Hormonal-Based Depression

Black cohosh (*Actaea racemosa*) is commonly used for depression that begins during puberty or associated with menstruation. The depression is deep with a "doom and gloom" component, and is often accompanied by muscle spasms, aches, and pains. Black cohosh's defining characteristic is the beautiful, light racemes on top of the plant but then deep, gnarled roots under the earth. Dr. Low Dog chooses this herb for the woman who reflects the characteristic of the plant: put together on the outside but an emotional mess on the inside. It is sold by Nature's Way as a whole root extract at 540 mg capsules (the bottle with the green cap and label) and also by Nature's Way as 40 mg of the standardized extract, 2.5 percent triterpene glycosides (the bottle with the purple cap). Take 1 capsule twice daily of either product.

Night blooming cereus (*Selenicereus grandifloras*). This plant is a beautiful night-blooming cactus. The fresh stem is the part used medicinally. It is especially good for depression mixed with anxiety expressed as excessive fear. It is very useful when combined with black cohosh. You can find it in an alcohol-free extract from www.hawaiipharm.com or as an alcohol tincture at the same website. Take 1 full dropper in 2–4 ounces of water and drink up to four times a day.

Bupleurum/Chai hu (*Bupleurum chinensis*). This herb is useful for liver qi stagnation. What is liver qi stagnation you might ask? It is a concept in Chinese medicine that reflects the stress and tension of modern life leading to symptoms of depression, moodiness, feeling wound-up, alternations of moods, intense frustration, anxiety, and irritability. Bupleurum is an excellent liver protector and support. It is rarely used alone but is commonly used with other herbs. Available from Hawaii Pharm as an alcohol-free glycerite extract. Follow the directions on the bottle.

Tiger lily (*Lilium tigrinum*). Tiger lily is a beautiful orange flower with spots. It is well-respected in traditional uses for the support of the female reproductive system, and David Winston uses it in conjunction with black cohosh to address the depression associated with menopause. This is a product that is not commercially available but could be made for you by a community herbalist. The dose would depend on how it is made.

Hypothyroid-Induced Depression

Bacopa (*Bacopa monnieri*). Also known as water hyssop or Brahmi, bacopa has been used in Ayurvedic medicine for centuries to relieve anxiety and improve cognition. It has beautiful white flowers and is a creeping herb found in wetlands. In a study with mice, high doses were shown to increase the amount of thyroxin (the main hormone produced by the thyroid) in the circulation.[4] It has been shown in studies to improve depression, anxiety, and cognitive performance. Himalaya makes a 750 mg caplet. When you get into the higher doses it becomes a stimulating herb, so be mindful of the dosage. Take one daily, preferably in the morning. Personally, I find this herb to be very effective.[5]

Red ginseng (*Panax [Asian] ginseng*). Ginseng has been used in Asian medicine for centuries and is highly prized. The natural color of ginseng root is white, the red color is the result of heating the root. Heating the root changes the biochemistry and the root becomes more stimulating and warming. The red ginseng is used for elders who are cold and slow—signs of hypothyroidism. It is warming, stimulating, and improves cognition as well as overall energy. Take as a tea, a tincture, or a capsule. Since it is a root, the tea has to be made by simmering 1–2 teaspoons of ground ginseng root in 12 ounces of water for 30 minutes, then letting it steep for another hour. Drink 2 cups daily. If taken as a tincture, the recommended dosage is 1 dropperful 3–4 times a day. Also available in capsule form. Take two 400–500 mg capsules of powdered herb or extract daily.[6, 7]

Bladderwrack (*Fucus vesiculosus*). Bladderwrack is a seaweed that is high in iodine and selenium. It has been used to improve hypothyroidism due to iodine deficiency. The movement in the general public toward sea salt consumption gives us a more complex set of minerals, but sea salt does not have iodine in sufficient quantities to maintain normal thyroid levels in humans. Therefore, bladderwrack can be a helpful supplement. This is a food taken best in soups or chewed directly. The dose is 1–2 teaspoons per day in food.[8]

Damiana (*Turnera diffusa*). Damiana is a shrub that grows in Mexico and southern California. It is widely served as a tea, a common beverage for men, women, and children in Mexico. It is well known there for its seemingly contradictory calming and stimulating effects. It is said to have aphrodisiac properties but since it is served to children, I doubt that. David Winston uses this for depression associated with hypothyroidism and combines it with Bacopa and Ashwagandha. Nature's Way sells a 400 mg capsule; the recommended dosage is 2 capsules three times a day. Damiana is also available in tea and tincture form. Do not use in pregnancy or lactation.

Hypothalamic-Pituitary Axis-Cortisol Regulation

Eleuthero (*Eleutherococcus senticosus*, *Synonym Acanthopanax senticosus*). Eleuthero is an adaptogen, the herb category that helps the body adapt to stress and is a modulator. Winston uses this herb for those who work hard, play hard, and hardly sleep. These are people who are stressed out, type A personalities. With this stress there is an increase in cortisol levels. This herb is the safest for long-term use. Dr. Low Dog reports that it blunts cortisol releasing hormone at the level of the hypothalamus. It is available as tincture, capsule, and dried herb root. The tea is made by simmering 1–2 teaspoons of herb per 12–16 ounces of water for 20–30 minutes and then steep for an hour. Drink up to 3 cups daily. The supplement dose will vary depending on the preparation—whole root, dried root, or extract. Follow the directions on the bottle of the product you choose. Good brands are Nature's Way, GAIA herbs, and Hawaii pharm. There is some adulteration in the marketplace, so it is important to purchase from a reputable company. The company should be able to tell you where the herb came from and have control over it from harvest to product.

American ginseng (*Panax quinquefolius*). American ginseng is not as well-known a plant in America as the Asian variety. Its characteristics are quite different from Asian ginseng in that it is cooler and not indicated for warming the cold person. Interestingly, American ginseng has been widely cultivated in the Americas, used by American Indian tribes traditionally and is exported to China where it is very popular in Chinese medicine. David Winston, in his book *Adaptogens: Herbs for Strength, Stamina and Stress Relief,* describes how he uses it to reduce stress levels, improve sleep, and balance an overstressed nervous system. These patients are burned out, have dark circles under their eyes, and are chronically fatigued. He believes it is best for the middle-aged person (defined as 40–60) who is feeling their strength and endurance waning. It is endangered as a wild herb, so purchase herbs labeled "organic woods-grown American ginseng." It is available as the herb, as a tincture, or as a capsule. As a capsule, take 500 mg twice a day. As an herb simmer for 20 minutes and then steep for half an hour. Take 4 ounces three times a day. The herb is available at www.mountainroseherbs.com and other online herb stores. This herb is very safe.

Schisandra (*Schisandra chinensis*). Known as five-flavored fruit, schisandra supports all the yin organs of the body. The yin organs are the nourishing and tonifying organs that support health: the liver, heart, spleen, lungs, and kidneys. Schisandra is used when there is a lack of physical and mental energy, as is common in depression. It helps improve concentration and yet reduces anxiety. It is available as a tincture, capsule, as the berry or as powder. You can purchase it from www.mountainroseherbs.com or www.starwest-botanicals.com. The recommended dose for the tincture is 2–4 ml, three to four times per day. For the tea, put 1–2 teaspoons of dried berries in 8–10 ounces of water, simmer for 5–10 minutes, and steep for 20–30 minutes. Each person will perceive one of the flavors more boldly than the others. Take 4 ounces three times daily. Capsule dose is 400–500 mg capsules, two to three times per day.

Hypothalamus-Pituitary-Adrenal Axis: Elevated Cortisol

When the body is stressed, cortisol, made by the adrenal gland, is secreted and the cortisol level in the body rises. When the stress becomes chronic, the cortisol levels remain high, and the type of depression experienced then is called a melancholic depression or depressed mood in light of high cortisol levels. This type of depression is often experienced along with a fair amount of anxiety. The herbs used to improve this type of depression manage the anxious component and are described in detail in the anxiety chapter in the next section.

Following are the herbs most often used to reduce cortisol.

Chamomile (*Anthemis mobilis*) and (*Matricaria recutita*). This is a common herb probably well-known to the reader as an herb to use for relaxation. It can also be used for depression with anxiety.

Lemon balm (*Melissa officianalis*). This herb is well known for its pleasant lemon flavor, fragrance, and uplifting effect.

Linden flowers (*Tilia europea*). Sold in Europe as a beverage and most known for its calming effects, especially with children.

St. John's wort (*Hypericum perforatum*). St. John's wort is a well-known and widely used herb and may be familiar to the reader. It has the reputation of being an anti-depressant.

Wild oats: (*Avena fatua, A. sativa*). Christopher Hobbs describes the use of this plant as a nerve support that is specific for the exhaustion due to depression. It may also be helpful for withdrawal from addictions.

Cardiovascular Depression

Jiaogulan (*Gynostemma pentaphyllum*). This herb in the gourd-cucumber family is relatively obscure in Western literature. The herb grows in southern China, Korea, and Japan, and I know of an herb school in the northwest mountains of North Carolina that grows it as well. It grows as a vine. The known constituents are called gypenosides and of the eighty-four identified, four are identical to the ginsenosides (the active ingredient in ginseng) found in Asian ginseng. Therefore,

Jiaogulan shares some of the same properties of Asian ginseng. In studies, Jiaogulan has shown to improve immune function and is an excellent detoxification herb. It was first brought to the attention of the Chinese government when many centenarians were identified in the province where Jiaogulan grows and is commonly consumed. Due to its ability to improve cardiac function, lipid, and blood sugar regulation, Jiaogulan is especially helpful for cardiac-induced depression. The dried herb is called the "Immortality Tea" due to the belief that this herb can extend life. You will find supplements of the Gynostemma root but to my knowledge and research there is no reason to consume the root. It is the leaf of the plant that is made into a tea and consumed. I recommend only consuming the capsules that provide extracts standardized to the gypenosides. Follow the directions on the bottle.

Hawthorn (*Crataegus spp.*). When I think of the cardiovascular contribution to depression, the first herb that comes to my mind is Hawthorn. Hawthorn is thought to be an alterative, an herb that is nourishing to the system. Dr. Sharol Marie Tilgner describes Hawthorn as an herb indicated for emotional heartache and to open oneself to forgiveness of self or others. Hawthorn is an herb that would be recommended in conjunction with others (Jiaogulan, for example) for the treatment of the underlying cardiovascular contribution to a depressed mental state. Hawthorn leaves and berries as a mixture is effective. To make a tea, simmer 1–2 teaspoons of herb in 8–10 ounces of water for 15 minutes and strain. Drink 4–8 ounces three times a day. It is also available in capsule form as a mixture of the berries, leaves, and flowers. The herb is available from www.mountainroseherbs.com, www.starwest-botanicals.com,

Bulk Herb store, Frontier Herbs, and others. If purchased as a capsule, follow the directions on the bottle. Gaia herbs makes a good product. It is also available as a solid extract, made by Alchemist and Herbalist. The solid extract has the consistency of a jam and is delicious. You can find it online at www.alchemist-herbalist.com and other online retailers.

Night blooming cereus. See above.

Rhodiola (*Rhodiola rosea*). Also known as arctic root, Rhodiola is used as an anti-depressant in the northern latitudes of Canada, Scandinavia, and Siberia. This lovely rose-shaped plant is helpful for mood regulation and has a long history of being used for the enhancement of physical and mental performance. It is very well studied by the Russian government and is given to their Olympic athletes. It is only in the last thirty years that Rhodiola has come into prominence in the United States because prior to that all the studies were published in Russian, Swedish, German, or Chinese. According to David Winston, Rhodiola is stimulating but not nourishing. It is second to Asian Ginseng in stimulating effects. It is the stimulating effects of Rhodiola that make it useful for depression. One would wonder if it caused anxiety, and in some patients, it does. UCLA however, in an open study, showed benefit in generalized anxiety disorder. The day after I read about that study, I had two patients tell me that they thought Rhodiola lessened their anxiety. Rhodiola is very drying, so a side effect can be dry mouth. The plant is available as a capsule. Be sure to buy the extract standardized to 3 percent rosavins and 1 percent salidrosides. Take 500 mg one to two times daily. Other herbalists recommend up to 1000–2000 mg, three times daily. It is also available in extract form.

Stroke-Induced Depression

Bacopa monnieri and Rosemary (*Rosmarinus offici-nalis*). See above.

Holy basil, Tulsi (*Ocimum tenuiflorum,* [*synonym O. sanctum*] *and O. gratissimum*). This herb grows naturally in the lowlands of India, in Sri Lanka, Pakistan, Myanmar, southern China, Thailand, and Malaysia. It is cultivated in gardens for daily use as a spice in cooking. It is considered sacred in Ayurvedic medicine, as it is considered a highly nourishing herb bringing health and longevity to the person who consumes it daily. It is known to have anti-depressant and anxiolytic properties. As is the case with so many of the herbs, it is used for a variety of ailments including gastrointestinal distress, coughs, bug bites, and stings. David Winston uses holy basil to enhance cerebral circulation along with the other herbs described above with the same indication such as bacopa, rosemary, and gingko biloba, an herb well-known to enhance cerebral blood flow. He finds it helpful to lessen the brain fog due to excessive marijuana smoking and to improve recovery from head trauma (including stroke). Tulsi is available as a dried herb, in teabags, as tablets, or as a tincture. For the tea, place a teaspoon of the herb in 8 ounces of boiling water and steep, covered for 5–10 minutes. Drink 4 ounces one to three times per day. If purchased as a capsule, be sure to buy something that is standardized to 2 percent ursolic acid. Follow the directions on the bottle. Holy basil is often added to other herbal products. Do not take in pregnancy.

Dr. Sharol Marie Tilgner is a naturopathic physician and nationally known speaker. She is the author of *Herbal Medicine from the Heart of the Earth* and has produced two herbal videos: *Edible and Medicinal Herbs,* Volumes I and II. She recommends the following anti-depressant formula.

Dr. Tilgner's Anti-depressant formula

St. John's wort *Hypericum perforatum*   25–40%

Eleuthero *Eleutherococcus senticosus*   15–20%

Skullcap *Scutellaria lateriflora*   5–20%

Schisandra *Schisandra chinensis*   10–20%

Oats-green *Avena sativa*   10–20%

Chamomile *Matricaria recutita*   5–10%

Rosemary *Rosmarinus officinalis*   5–10%

Lavender essential oil *Lavandula officinalis* 1–2 drops per ounce

Orange essential oil *Citrus aurantium*   1–2 drops per ounce

If this is made as an extract: for acute symptoms take 30–70 drops in a little water three to four times per day, and for restorative effects take 30–50 drops in a little water, two to three times per day.

This can also be made as a tea. Say you want to make 10 cups of tea. You would need to use 10 teaspoons of herbs and 10 cups of water. Follow the ratios above. For instance, use 2.5 teaspoons of St. John's wort, 1.5 teaspoons of Eleuthero, ½ teaspoon of Scutellaria, and so on.

Caution: Do not use in pregnancy. Indicated for mild to moderate depression.

Please remember to seek professional advice for any mental health condition.

4

THE GUT-BRAIN CONNECTION

first learned about the gut-brain connection ten or more years ago. It was a novel idea then, but now it has worked its way into mainstream thinking. I have patients that come into the office asking about it. Many of you may know about it and wonder how it applies to psychiatry.

Why should you care about bowel health if you suffer with depression or anxiety? Because bowel health has a direct effect on the brain. The brain manages our relationships in a similar way that the gut manages our nutrition. When the boundaries of the gut are healthy, it knows what nutrients to allow into the bloodstream and what is toxic and should not be allowed.

The brain makes that same assessment with our relationships. When our relationship boundaries are clear, we know what to do with other people. We get to know people (digest the relationship), decide who to bring close (absorb into the bloodstream), who is toxic, and who needs to be kept out of our lives (excreted from the body).

As a psychiatrist, working on gut health is one of the more important and frequent things that I do. If there were such a thing as professional reincarnation I would come back as a gastroenterologist.

The gastrointestinal disorders that I treat as a psychiatrist are constipation, irritable bowel syndrome, and most importantly "leaky gut," or in medical terms, hyperpermeability syndrome. When most people think about the "gut" they are thinking colon, or large bowel. Certainly, colonics have existed for centuries to improve health, and there has been a strong focus on colon health for a long time. However, the part of the bowel that is leaky is the small bowel. It is in the small bowel where most of the absorption of nutrients takes place.

There are anatomical, enzymatic, and hormonal connections between the brain and the gastrointestinal tract. In my years of practicing psychiatry, almost everyone who suffers with depression or anxiety has gastrointestinal distress of some type. People who are anxious often have gastrointestinal upset to go with it; sometimes it is vomiting, sometimes diarrhea. There are some people who have terrible constipation. The gastrointestinal symptoms can be debilitating, but at the very least they are distressing. It is also not uncommon for irritable bowel syndrome to be found alongside premenstrual syndrome. The premenstrual symptoms and the bowel symptoms often come together. You can imagine how uncomfortable someone would be with the emotionality of the premenstrual symptoms and the irritability in the gastrointestinal system simultaneously.

The Digestive System

To begin to talk about how the brain and the gut interact we need to take a trip through the digestive system. Digestion is a bit complicated, so hang in there with me. I promise I will tie it back to the brain.

Before you read on, ask yourself the questions, Where does digestion begin? Where do you think food is digested first?

Digestion actually begins in the mouth. This is the reason chewing is important. Dr. John Christopher, a renowned naturopath (many of his lectures are free on YouTube), taught me how to chew my food. Now, most of you think you already know how to chew your food.

Dr. Christopher recommends that you chew your solid food until it liquefies before swallowing it. (I have since learned that this recommendation was something he learned from *Back to Eden* by Jethro Kloss.) Many of you may have heard of the importance of chewing food, but to chew it enough to liquify it before swallowing was new to me. I make this recommendation for good gut health, but also to those who want to lose weight. It is so simple that it feels silly. But it is effective. When I implemented the process of chewing food to liquify it, I went from the fastest eater at the table to the slowest. I found I could identify and enjoy many more flavors, and I was inspired to begin cooking with more spices. I also noticed that I felt full and satisfied much more quickly, so I actually did not want to eat as much. My bite sizes became smaller. Without intending to lose weight, I lost weight. Just from chewing my solid food to liquid. Chewing your food thoroughly like that also keeps you from emotionally, mindlessly eating. For those of you who are emotional eaters, chewing your food until it becomes liquid will slow you down and can be very challenging when you are upset or extremely busy.

Why is chewing so important?

The goal of digestion is to take large chunks of food and break it down into molecular-sized particles that will be able to cross a cell membrane and become nutrients for our body to use. Think of a piece of broccoli. It is thick, fibrous, and much too large to cross a cell membrane. After digestion the broccoli is made into molecules of nutrients that can cross the gut cell membranes and enter the bloodstream to be used as the body needs it.

The act of chewing prepares the body for digestion. It turns on all the mechanisms contained within the digestive tract that allow us to take food and turn it into nutrients. The saliva starts the process of breaking down food, then passes it on to the stomach. The stomach does its part in breaking things down by secreting acid and by mechanical pressure. This is an area that is affected by anxiety. The sphincter that is supposed to keep food in the stomach sometimes allows stomach acid to go up into the esophagus, contributing to heartburn. Heartburn and gastritis are commonly found along with anxiety and depression. Treating both the stomach and the mood issues is more effective than addressing one alone. Both can be treated with non-medication approaches such as herbal remedies, diet, and lifestyle modifications.

The stomach passes the partially digested food into the small bowel, which continues the breakdown process. The small bowel gets help from the pancreas and gall bladder, which send enzymes into the bowel to help break things down. You may notice that digestive enzymes sold as supplements are pancreatic enzymes (chymotrypsin, amylase, lipase, and others). This is why they are needed in the small bowel to help with digestion. The liver sends in its support, too, by sending in bile. This is one of the reasons so many supplements and gut health recommendations include liver cleanses or liver supports such as ox bile.

It is interesting to note that in Asian and ancient Greek medicine, the bile is important emotionally. In those systems, the liver is the source of anger and melancholy; bilious people are ones who are ill-tempered and generally disagreeable. It is common for people who have depression to be ill-tempered and might be considered "bilious."

The majority of digestion happens in the small bowel, which is in close contact with the bloodstream and the immune system. The cells of the walls of the small bowel are tightly held together by junctions. The purpose of the tight junctions is to keep the contents of the bowel in the bowel unless the cell decides that the nutrient is appropriate to be absorbed into the bloodstream. If the cells of the gut wall become inflamed, say from chronic stress or poor nutrition, the tight junctions open and there is movement from the contents of the gut to the bloodstream. This is what is meant by the wall being "leaky."

There are specialized areas of immune cells located in the small bowel called Peyer's patches, so the gut is our first line of defense against infection. The contents of the small bowel have direct contact with the immune system here. This is a good thing if you have a serious infection. However, when stress and anxiety open the gut wall many components of the gut contents can pass into the bloodstream. Our immune system then reacts to the bowel contents and we can develop autoimmune diseases and allergies. The barrier between self and non-self has become compromised.

The next step in the digestive process takes place in the

colon. The gut contents, now greatly digested, pass into the final stage of digestion. What happens in the colon is largely the absorption of water and the excretion of waste and toxins. If too much water is absorbed, there is constipation; if too little water is absorbed there is diarrhea. The colon is also the place where bacteria is prevalent. The bacteria located in the colon break down the intestinal contents in a fermentation process. The bacterial activity makes vitamin K, vitamin B12, and short-chain fatty acids that we need but cannot make ourselves. These are absorbed in the colon, along with water. The bacterial activity found in the colon (and small bowel) is very important to health. The bacterial constitution of the colon is what is referred to as the microbiome. The microbiome sets the stage for vitamin absorption, the excretion of toxins, and interaction with the immune system.

The function of the microbiome is so important that the microbiome of the mother's body makes a difference in the child's immune system. Research has shown that improving the bacterial health of the mother before delivery and the baby after delivery can markedly reduce the risk of atopic dermatitis (eczema), an allergic hyper-reactivity. Having a comprehensive microbiome improves the overall immune function of the body and reduces inflammation in the gut and the brain as well as the body as a whole.

Let me summarize the sequence of events that leads us from eating food to inflammation of the brain and body.

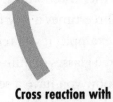

**Digested food
and stress**

**Open tight junctions
in the small bowel wall**

**Fragments enter blood
and get picked up by
immune cells**

**Cross reaction with
other tissues of
the body**

**Inflammation in the brain
and psychiatric symptoms
and autoimmune
disorders**

Sequence of events.

Figure 4.1
Diagram by Dr. Lillian Somner.

This is why, as a psychiatrist, I spend a lot of time talking to people about their diet and how to lessen the inflammation in the intestinal tract—all with the intent of improving their psychiatric symptoms. The first step to reducing the inflammation in the brain is to reduce the inflammation in the gut. The process I just described is called the gut-brain axis and is modulated through the hypothalamic-pituitary-adrenal (HPA) axis. More on the HPA axis later.

So how do you reduce inflammation in the gut?

The first step in reducing gut inflammation is removing those things that are causing inflammation. An elimination diet is a good place to start. A simple one is to remove the following foods from your diet for three weeks: eggs, dairy, gluten (all wheat products, thickeners, salad dressings), sugar, processed meats, corn (including corn syrups), and alcohol. After three weeks, add one item into the diet. Add that item in three times a day for three days and see if symptoms return. For example, if you remove all items and reintroduce dairy, drink three glasses of milk daily for three days. If symptoms return you know you have a sensitivity to dairy and should avoid it. If you choose to add gluten back in, eat three slices of bread a day for three days. If you have any symptoms or discomfort, you should avoid gluten. If you have no symptoms after the three days, then you are probably able to tolerate the food. Keep adding in the removed foods to determine all that you have a sensitivity to, and permanently remove those foods from your diet for the sake of your gut.

This simple dietary change can make a very big difference. I will give you an example. I was treating my patient Rod with transcranial magnetic stimulation (TMS), the magnetic treatment of medication-resistant depression. The treatment requires going into the clinic to receive the magnetic stimulation five days a week for six weeks. This was the second time he was receiving the treatment series. The first time he missed half his sessions because of diarrhea that kept him from leaving the house. He missed his first scheduled appointment with me for the same reason. When I did see him, I asked him about his symptoms and recommended that he try the elimination diet. He agreed and was able to find the source of his gut issue. He did not miss another appointment and was able to attend all the TMS treatments. When I asked him what he had removed he told me it was dairy. Now that he was dairy free, he could leave the house freely. He also had a very good response to the TMS treatment.

The second step to reduce gut inflammation is to actually repair the gut. In this case, repair means to not only reduce the inflammation in the intestinal wall but to also tighten up the tight junctions that have loosened to prevent continued leakage of the intestinal contents. It may also require reducing the small bowel overgrowth either with medication or herbs.

There are many herbs that are helpful in repairing the gut. I always recommend using the herbal treatments for three months to get the best benefit. What follows is a list of herbs to choose from. I am listing here herbs that are easy to use, easy to find, and effective. There are many others and a trained herbalist or physician with herbal training can make specific recommendations for your particular case. Be sure to seek appropriate medical attention for any gastrointestinal problems. There is no substitute for appropriate medical care.

Marshmallow (*Althea officinalis*). Marshmallow is a mucilaginous herb that will help repair the mucous layer of the epithelium of the intestine. The mucous layer gets damaged from the inflammation and irritation of high levels of stress, highly processed foods, allergies, and infections. The mucous layer is a critical participant in protection of the gut wall and also gives the probiotics (the healthy bacteria described below) a place to take hold. If this layer is damaged, it is more difficult to establish the healthy microbiota.

When there is upper GI distress take marshmallow as a cold infused drink. Put a teaspoon of the chopped root in a glass of water and let it sit overnight. Strain and drink on an empty stomach. The more water you have the less gelatinous the drink will be. If you use a small amount of water, it will be the consistency of porridge. It is still useable in the thicker form, just not as pleasant. When there is lower GI distress, take marshmallow as a capsule and take with food. The food will push the marshmallow into the lower bowel where it will soothe the gut. Do this daily until symptoms have cleared. It may take up to three months. Marshmallow is available by Nature's Way as a capsule and you can also find it as a cut and sifted herb. I do not recommend the powder form. When there is acute gastritis, the relief after drinking marshmallow tea is very rapid, within minutes. This is a personal favorite.

Peppermint (*Mentha piperita L.*). Peppermint as an essential oil, which is enteric coated so it is not absorbed in the stomach but goes farther into the intestine, is considered first line treatment for irritable bowel syndrome. The enteric-coated products are often mixed with essential oil of caraway, which is an excellent choice as it reduces bloating and gas. The dose is usually 0.2 ml of each oil per capsule. Take one before each meal to avoid intestinal cramping. An excellent product is Regimint. It can be purchased at www.regimint.com or from your favorite vendor.

Licorice root extract (*Glycyrrhiza glabra* or *Glycyrrhiza uralensis*). The Latin name of licorice root means sweet root, and the root does have a sweet taste. Taking a dose of licorice before a meal can be helpful for digestion. However, because licorice contains glycyrrhizin, which can raise the blood pressure, hold sodium, and excrete potassium, I recommend limiting your consumption of the whole root to a maximum of

600 mg daily, which gives you a safe amount of glycyrrhizin. If you are concerned about the potential of hypertension, an alternative is deglycyrrhizinated licorice (DGL). DGL must be chewed and is best consumed before each meal and before bed to prevent early morning gastritis. The potency of DGL is less than that of licorice root but it is still very helpful for gut repair.

Do not take licorice if you are pregnant.

Turmeric (*Curcuma longa*). This root is most widely known for the anti-inflammatory effects of the active compound, curcumin. Curcumin is commonly sold over the counter in supplement form with some type of black pepper product, most commonly BioPerine (Piperine). The pepper extract is needed to enhance the absorption of curcumin into the bloodstream. If you are using curcumin as an anti-inflammatory for the intestine, then you do *not* want it to be absorbed. It needs to remain in the gut. Therefore, you may take it directly as a spice from your kitchen. You need a minimum of 1200 mg of curcumin daily. There is approximately 200 mg of curcumin in a teaspoon of turmeric. Take 6 teaspoons daily, mixed in food. Divide it up so you do not take it all at once. It can upset your stomach and cause some gastrointestinal irritation if taken in too high a dose. Another option is to take it as a standardized extract. The amount of curcumin needed is 1200 mg daily.

Do not take if pregnant or if you have active gall bladder disease.

Chamomile (*Matricaria recutita*). Chamomile is a delicious tea, safe for young and old. It has been used for colic in newborns and can be used for elders with gastrointestinal distress. It is an excellent anti-inflammatory and also is a nervine, causing some relaxation. A nice way to make the tea is as a cold

infusion. Put a teabag of chamomile in a cup of room temperature water and let it steep. Drink it cool. It can also be served
hot with a little honey if desired. Drink 1–2 cups daily, or when-
ever the stomach is upset. Chamomile is in the ragweed family.
Do not use if there is an allergic reaction to ragweed or other
plants in that family.

Healing the Gut, Step 2

The next step in reducing gut inflammation is to replace the
constitution of the microbiome of the gut. The best way to do
this is with the use of probiotics and prebiotics. There are several probiotics and prebiotics available over the counter. Probiotics are the bacteria that are "friendly," that help us make
our vitamins, that take up room so "bad" bacteria cannot have
a place to live. Most people have heard about probiotics and
many are confused because there are so many to choose from.
We'll talk more about probiotics below.

Prebiotics, such as inulin, oligofructose, arabinogalactans,
and others, feed the probiotic. There are herbal sources of prebiotics. For example, dandelion and burdock root are high in
the prebiotic, inulin. These can be eaten as food in the diet.
Chicory, a bitter green found in many cuisines, is another food
source of prebiotics. It is also high in inulin.

Let's take a closer look at probiotics. Most of us have taken
antibiotics when sick. Antibiotics kill off pathogenic bacteria.
Probiotics, on the other hand, introduce non-toxic, live bacteria
to the gut. Before antibiotics existed, the probiotic would be
used to treat a gastrointestinal infection by replacing the pathogenic bacteria with a beneficial one. (This is still done today in
those whose microbiome is not able to maintain health by way

of a fecal transplant.) A probiotic is defined as bacteria that is not harmful to the body but is helpful in reducing inflammation, protecting against infection, and that makes our vitamin K and vitamin B12. However, the main purpose of probiotics is to improve food assimilation via fermentation. Fermentation is the process by which nutrients are removed from the food we eat and absorbed.

Common Probiotics

- *Lactobacillus rheuteri*
- *Lactobacillus rhamnosus*
- *Lactobacillus casei*
- *Bifidobacterium infantis*
- Other *Bifidobacterium* species
- *Saccharomyces* species

Taking a probiotic supplement, especially if it has some prebiotic contained within it, can be beneficial to reducing the inflammation in the gut and the body. Having a healthy microbiome can help reduce allergy by calming the immune responses to particles found in the environment.

How do you choose a probiotic? What do all those designations mean? A probiotic is a bacterium with a first and last name and some identifying numbers. The first name is the genus, the second name is the species, and the third identifying letters and numbers is the strain. For example, L. acidophilus SD 5212 means the genus is Lactobacillus, the species is acidophilus, and the strain is SD 5212. When research is done on the probiotic to test it for efficacy and survivability, the bacteria are researched based on their strain. The reason the strain is included is that the entire species may not be useful.

Probiotics are sold over the counter in colony forming units (CFUs). Bacteria grow in colonies, hence the measurement of colony forming units. Bifidobacterium and Lactobacillus are the strains most commonly found in over-the-counter supplements. I recommend probiotics that contain the following species: *Lactobacillus rheuteri*, *Lactobacillus casei*, and *Bifidobacterium infantis*, as well as other Bifidobacterium species. *Lactobacillus rhamnosus* has been very well studied but is only available as Culturelle, sold over the counter. Saccharomyces species may also be included and are a good adjunct, although they are not a bacterium. The Saccharomyces species can be very helpful for preventing the development of *Clostridium deficile* colitis following antibiotic treatment and the consequent development of irritable bowel syndrome. The amount of CFUs needed to be beneficial varies from species to species. Most commercially available products are proprietary, and you will not know how much of each strain is in the product. Therefore, I can only make a general recommendation that the probiotic has a complement of as many of the strains listed above as possible. There should also be at least 80 billion CFUs.

The bottom line is that healing the gut is of the utmost importance in treating mental illness, for a damaged gut can lead to inflammation in the brain and psychiatric symptoms. Changing one's diet and adding the right herbs and supplements can heal inflammation in the gut, close the tight junctions, and improve the microbiome—resulting in a healthy gut and healthy brain.

5

THE CORTISOL CONNECTION

We all experience stress in our lives. How our bodies and mind manage that stress determines how we feel on a day-to-day basis.

Dr. Hans Selye, whose life's work was studying the biological effects of stress, developed the first model of the stress reaction. He defined three phases of stress. The first phase is the acute phase—when stress is an insult to the body, be it an infection or fever or an interpersonal upset. The second phase is the resistance phase. This phase is one in which the person is able to manage the stress but struggles with it over a long period of time; in this case the stressor is chronic. The resistance phase can last for months to years depending on the constitution of the individual. The final phase is the exhaustion phase. This phase is when the body begins to lose its resiliency and it is not uncommon for the person to become ill.

Stress is modulated through the hypothalamic-pituitary-adrenal system (HPA axis). The HPA axis is very important for the regulation of stress reactions in the body. Cortisol is the stress hormone that is responsible for managing our physical response to stress and has a profound effect on our mood and our energy level. The physiological management of stress is done by cortisol.

Let's look at how the HPA axis works and how it regulates stress. The HPA axis describes the interaction between the hypothalamus (H), pituitary gland (P), and the adrenal gland (A). The hypothalamus and the pituitary are located in the brain. The adrenal gland is located on top of the kidney. When something stressful happens, our sympathetic nervous system immediately releases epinephrine and norepinephrine, which activate the typical stress/fear responses, like an increased heartbeat and perspiration. About ten seconds later, the HPA axis kicks in. The hypothalamus releases corticotropin-releasing hormone (CRH), which increases the activity of the sympathetic nervous system and tells the pituitary gland to release adrenocorticotropic hormone (ACTH). The ACTH travels through the bloodstream down to the adrenal glands and binds to the outer surfaces of the glands, activating the adrenals to release more hormones, including cortisol. The brain perceives the need for cortisol and tells the adrenal gland what to do. The adrenal gland secretes cortisol, or adrenaline. The cortisol allows the body to respond to stress in the acute phase. In the resistance phase, the cortisol level may still be high, but the body is struggling. In the exhaustion phase the cortisol levels drop. It is in this particular phase that the body feels exhausted, wiped out, vulnerable to illness. When the person moves into the exhaustion phase the person feels that they have "crashed."

Phase 1: Acute Phase	Phase 2: Resistance	Phase 3: Exhaustion
Appropriate response to a normal stress	Stress is chronic, person struggles but is able to hold on	No juice left, vulnerable to becoming ill
Cortisol rises and then falls	Cortisol is chronically high	Cortisol levels drop

Having high cortisol levels affects the entire body. There is sleep disruption with early morning awakening. Serotonin and dopamine levels drop, leading to depressed mood and lack of pleasure. You have an increased risk for cardiovascular disease, as high cortisol promotes the buildup of plaque deposits in the arteries. There is also an increased risk of infection. Cortisol puts the immune system on high alert, and after prolonged high levels the immune system becomes overwhelmed, leaving the body vulnerable to infection. If the gut is "leaky" and some colonic contents are in the bloodstream, they also contribute to the immune system's over-activity.

The cortisol source of depression is not routinely identified in conventional psychiatry, but it is a useful and important diagnosis to make. In my psychiatric residency I was not taught to measure the cortisol levels or that the cortisol levels were important. Now I make sure to measure cortisol levels in the body. A saliva test is a good way to do this. Cortisol levels vary normally throughout the day. If the levels are elevated at night the person is less likely to sleep well. If elevated in the early morning the person may have awakened early and starts the day with anxiety.

The following chart shows some herbs that are commonly used to lower cortisol and how they interact with the HPA axis.

Herbal Remedy	What part of the HPA Axis is affected
Ashwagandha	Blunts ACTH at the level of the pituitary
Panax ginseng	Blunts ACTH at the level of the pituitary
Rhodiola	Blunts CRH at the level of the hypothalamus
Eleuthero	Blunts CRH at the level of the hypothalamus
L-theanine, an amino acid from green tea	Reduces catecholamine (the flight or fight neurotransmitters) release from the adrenal gland

There are several commercial products on the market that are available for lowering cortisol levels. They are known as calmatives. These are some of my favorites.

Name	Active Ingredients	Dosage
Metagenics Serenagen	Comprehensive herbal product using both Western and Chinese herbs	Take 2 daily
Dr. Amen's BrainMD Every Day Stress Relief	Relora (magnolia and philodendron), Holy Basil, Taurine, L-theanine	Take 4 daily
Orthomolecular Botanicalm	Kava rhizome, Chamomile flowers, Hops strobile, Passion flower, Valerian root	Take 1 daily

Name	Active Ingredients	Dosage
Phosphatidylserine (available from multiple vendors)	A fatty substance that covers and protects the cells in your brain and carries messages between them	Take 100 mg before bed to lessen morning anxiety

I also recommend a good multivitamin with minerals because vitamins C, B6, and K, as well as calcium, magnesium, and zinc, are all depleted with stress.

We have looked at what happens when the cortisol levels are too high, but sometimes the body can "crash" and go into what Dr. Selye referred to as the exhaustion phase. What happens then is that the body feels like it has run out of gas. The person feels like everything is overwhelming. They are not sleeping well, they are fatigued, low energy, they have no libido. In this state they can have more pain because the cortisol is not available as the anti-inflammatory. They can have allergies and autoimmune reactions.

There is no correlate to this in conventional medicine. The low cortisol response is known in the vernacular as adrenal fatigue, but is technically hypocortisolism. The depression that is associated with hypocortisolism is characterized by lethargy and fatigue and is considered atypical. When speaking to these patients you feel as though they are on their last nerve.

Let's look at some remedies for supporting the adrenals when they are reduced in function. I happen to be a fan of using the bovine extracts of the adrenal gland itself either alone or in conjunction with herbal preparations. A very good combination is the desiccated (dried) adrenal gland and licorice root extract. The licorice root extract will keep the cortisol around longer by inhibiting the enzyme that breaks it down, 11β-hydroxysteroid dehydrogenase. If you are cortisol depleted, then keeping the cortisol that you do have around longer can be advantageous. Working with a trained practitioner will help you decide what your cortisol levels are and how best to improve them.

Some of my favorite products are:

Name	Active Ingredients	Dosage
Metagenics Adreset	Cordyceps, Asian ginseng, *Rhodiola rosea*	Take 2 daily
Metagenics Licorice Plus	Licorice root extract, Ashwagandha, Herbal blend with *Rhemannia glutonosa*, Chinese yam (*Dioscorea oppositifolia*)	Take 1 daily
Thorne Cortex	Bovine adrenal cortex and whole adrenal extract, Licorice root extract, vitamin and mineral support	Take 1 daily
Thorne Adrenal Cortex	Desiccated bovine adrenal cortex	Take 1 to 2 daily
Klaire Labs Adrenal Cortex Concentrate	Desiccated bovine adrenal cortex concentrate	Take 1 daily

What I have observed over the years of practice is that practitioners who are not familiar with hypocortisolism may use stimulant medications to give the patient the energy that they lack. This is problematic, as it burns out the patient even further. It is better to identify the underlying problem and address the adrenal deficiency. When this is done the patient feels the difference. They feel nourished and they have more energy, but are not "wired up."

6

THE THYROID CONNECTION

Hormonal issues play a large role in depression. There are several hormones that have an impact on depressed mood. In this chapter, I will explain the role of the thyroid hormones. In the next chapter, we will take a look at the sex steroids—estrogen, progesterone, and testosterone. I also want to touch on vitamin D, and insulin, hormones rarely included in hormonal discussions of mood.

Thyroid

In July 2019, I attended the Hormone Advanced Practice Module presented by the Institute for Functional Medicine (IFM). There were a couple of fascinating take-aways from that module. The first take-away was that to treat the thyroid one should treat the adrenals first. Treating the adrenals first was always what I did and what colleagues of mine did, but it was not what was taught in medical school. That this protocol was becoming standard practice was a positive change. The second take-away was that the dysfunction of the hormonal system is a *reaction to* and *consequence of* lifestyle. Therefore, the first line treatment of hormonal dysfunction is lifestyle interventions.

It is fitting that I should discuss the importance of optimizing thyroid function to treat depression immediately following a discussion of evaluating the adrenal gland and its contribution to mental health. In the last chapter on the cortisol connection, I described how the cortisol level can be high and contribute to a melancholic depression or low and contribute to an atypical depression. As psychiatrists we examine the thyroid hormone in the case of depression, but it is a good idea to treat the adrenals first, before treating the thyroid. That way the body has the hormonal support to respond to thyroid interventions.

The concept that hormonal dysfunction is the *result* of life-style specifically stressful, toxic lifestyle was especially fascinating to me. It reminded me of the idea of a metabolic switch, identified by Dr. Dale Bredesen in the development of Alzheimer's disease. Dr. Bredesen has identified, through years of research, that lifestyle events such as poor-quality food, insulin resistance, infection, and brain injury cause metabolic insults to the brain. After so many insults, the metabolic switch flips and the brain develops amyloid plaques, which kill off brain cells and cognitive impairment begins. To reverse the Alzheimer's process then requires a reversal of those insults and the metabolic switch flips back to normal. The IFM presented something similar for the hormonal system. Although there may not be a specific switch as in the case of Alzheimer's disease, the idea is the same. We insult our hormonal system with the stressful, toxic lifestyle and it breaks down on us. When we remove those stressors and toxins, the hormonal system is able to click back on. It may be able to click back on enough to not require prescription hormones. However, if the system is too damaged, then prescription hormones will be needed.

Before we can talk about how the thyroid system goes awry,

we need to see how thyroid is made and what it does. The thyroid gland is considered to be the master gland because there are thyroid receptors everywhere in the body. Some signs of low thyroid are dry skin, constipation (hard stools with decreased frequency), fatigue, low mood, diffuse hair loss, cold intolerance, puffy face and hands. Hypothyroidism can also increase the low-density lipoproteins that contribute to vascular disease.

Thyroid production begins in the brain. Thyrotropin-releasing hormone (TRH) is produced in the hypothalamus and its job is to tell the anterior pituitary to release thyroid-stimulating hormone (TSH). TSH is released by the anterior pituitary and goes to the thyroid gland in the neck and tells the thyroid gland to make thyroid hormone. The thyroid hormone that is made is 95 percent T4, 5 percent T3. In the systemic circulation, T4 is converted to T3, a process that requires an adequate amount of cortisol. T3 is the most metabolically active form of thyroid hormone. T4 can also be converted to rT3, an inactive form of thyroid hormone. When rT3 is elevated, the thyroid function is ineffective.

When there is enough thyroid hormone circulating in the bloodstream, the thyroid hormone goes back to the anterior pituitary and tells it that no more TSH is needed. This is a negative feedback loop, keeping thyroid hormones in balance.

What are the insults to this system that interfere with how the thyroid works in the body? Stress is a big one. When we experience stress our CRH rises leading to a rise in the feeling of being stressed by way of increased cortisol. This lowers the TRH, which then leads to a lower TSH and a lower thyroid level in the body.

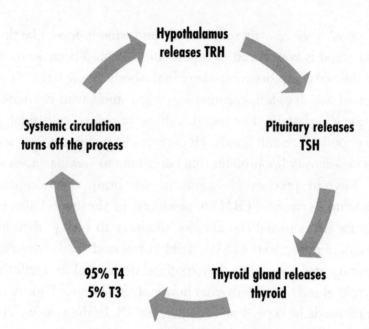

Figure 6.1

Diagram by Dr. Lillian Somner.

STRESS →Increased CRH→Increased cortisol
→Decreased TRH →Decreased TSH→
Decreased T3 and Increased conversion of T4 to rT3,
the inactive form of T3

This is how stress with increased cortisol can lead to hypo-thyroidism.

Subclinical hypothyroidism is something that happens as well. Subclinical hypothyroidism is when the T4 does not convert to T3 in spite of normal TSH levels. This often occurs when the cortisol level is low rather than high and the person is in a state of burnout. If there is an insufficient amount of cortisol, the body will not have the ability to make the conversion from T4 to T3. This is one reason it is important to assess and treat the cortisol levels first, before treating the thyroid.

Inflammation is a major player in reducing thyroid function.

Inflammation→Increases stress directly→Decreases TRH

Inflammation→IL10, TNF→Increases CRH →Decreases TSH

Inflammation→Increases ACTH→Decreases T4→T3

As I described in the prior chapter on the gastrointestinal system, systemic inflammation and autoimmune disorders often start in the gut and with the diet. One dietary correlation with hypothyroidism is celiac disease, also called celiac sprue, the autoimmune disease characterized by the inability to tolerate gluten. Symptoms include diarrhea and cramping, and usually celiac disease affects the small intestine so there is also marked nutritional deficiency. When there is evidence of celiac disease, check for autoimmune thyroiditis. There is a three-fold risk of autoimmune thyroiditis (Hashimoto's thyroiditis) in the presence of celiac disease. Changing the diet to improve inflammation and the hyperpermeability of the gut is of utmost importance in these cases.

Some nutritional deficiencies in celiac disease include iron, zinc, folic acid, vitamin B12, calcium, selenium, iodine, vitamins A, D, E and K. All of these are critical cofactors in the production of thyroid hormone. Supplementation of iron will improve the utilization of iodine for the production of thyroid hormone. Diets either high or low in iodine have an increased risk for Hashimoto's thyroiditis.

Even when celiac disease is not present, nutritional deficits may be present and may be a major player in hypothyroidism. The normal production of thyroid hormone requires an appropriate level of vitamin A, vitamin D (50–80 ng/ml ideally), and iron (measure ferritin, ideal greater than 50), as well as zinc, L-tyrosine, and iodine. Many people are deficient in these minerals and vitamins. Iodine deficiency is more common with the use of sea salt, which is not fortified with iodine.

Medications can also interfere with the conversion of T4 to T3. Common medications that interfere with thyroid conversion are listed below:

- Beta blockers, used to lower blood pressure and slow heart rate
- Birth control pills
- Estrogen replacement
- Lithium (which is why we follow thyroid function when lithium is prescribed)
- Phenytoin
- Theophylline
- Chemotherapy

Environmental toxins also affect the conversion of T4 to T3. Common heavy metals are cadmium (found in our air) and lead. These metals affect women more than men. There are more than 150 environmental toxins that can affect the thyroid.

If we have a reduction of thyroid function as a result of toxins it is important that our detoxification processes are in good condition. That means that the liver and the kidneys need to be working at optimal levels. One herb that is well known to support the liver is milk thistle (*Silybum marianum*). What is not as well known is that it is very effective for the support of the kidney as well. Often the same person will have trouble with both organs. Milk thistle is not well absorbed so the doses need to be high. It is very safe, with no drug-herb interactions. Milk thistle tea is completely ineffective, as no silymarin is water-soluble, therefore I do not recommend it.

If you have symptoms of hypothyroidism and if you have a thyroid-induced depression, *please* see a professional and take medication if necessary. If you are working with a functional medicine physician and are being monitored regularly, or if you have difficulty stabilizing your thyroid, you may benefit from nutritional supplementation and/or the herbs listed below. Research has shown them to improve hypothyroidism.

Herbs That Support Thyroid Function

Bladderwrack (*Fucus vesiculosus*). A common seaweed rich in minerals and trace elements. It contains potassium iodide. Put 1 to 2 teaspoons of the dried seaweed in 10 ounces of water. Simmer for 15 minutes and then let steep for half an hour. Take 4 ounces two to three times per day.

Bacopa monnieri. A stimulant for the thyroid. Take an oral supplementation of 1000 mg, once or twice daily. If using a tincture, take 2–3 ml, three times daily, of a 1:5 solution.

Stinging nettle (*Urtica dioica*). Has historically been used for the treatment of goiter. Take 1.5 to 2 ml of 1:5 tincture three times daily. Take 2–4 grams of dry herb three times a day.

Ashwagandha (*Withania somnifera*) has been used historically to improve thyroid function and has a high iron content. It has also been used for iron deficient anemia. To make as a tea, put 1–2 teaspoons of the herb in 12 ounces of water or almond milk. Simmer for 15 minutes. Steep for ½ hour. Take 4 ounces two or three times per day. Also available as an extract or in supplement form. Many people may not like the flavor of the tea. Contraindicated in pregnancy.

Supplements That Help Support Thyroid Function

- Selenium
- Zinc
- Vitamin D
- Vitamin A
- Iodine
- Iron
- Folic acid
- Vitamin B12
- Vitamin E
- Calcium
- Vitamin K
- Vitamins B2, B3, B6

A good multivitamin with minerals should provide you with an adequate amount of these nutrients.

Again, it's important to work with your health care practitioner. Be sure you get your thyroid levels measured and monitored on a regular basis.

7

THE SEX STEROID CONNECTION

When most people think about hormonal imbalance, they think about the sex steroid hormones: estrogen, progesterone, and testosterone. These are the hormones most familiar to the general public and most discussed on the Internet and in books. I want to spend some time here because it is an important topic. It is also a huge topic and way beyond the scope of this book.

What I would like to do, though, is discuss the common problems that I see as a psychiatrist. I find myself addressing painful menses, which can increase the stress and misery of a woman. I find myself treating premenstrual syndrome (PMS) or premenstrual dysphoric disorder (PMDD). One patient had such severe PMS that her family put her in a trailer on their property because she was too irritable to be around. How sad is that? I find myself treating depression that is a direct result of hormonal dysregulation and also depression associated with PMS.

Over the years I have developed a second sense about hormones. When I work with someone who is depressed, moody, anxious, and generally miserable, I expect that if I investigate the menstrual pattern I will find abnormalities, and I often do.

I have seen dermatologists treat adult acne with Spirono-lactone, a blood pressure medication used to treat polycystic ovary syndrome (PCOS). What is missing is the investigation into the hormonal disturbance that caused the acne in the first place. They don't measure testosterone or measure fasting insulin looking for insulin resistance. I think this is a disservice to the patient. When a woman presents with adult-onset acne, she should have blood work performed to rule out PCOS, and a discussion of PCOS and its consequences (infertility, insulin resistance, diabetes) should take place.

You may be wondering why a psychiatrist would be treating these conditions. It's because these conditions have a major impact on the psychic health of women. For some reason, these conditions are often left untreated and the woman is left to suffer.

Of course women's health is a big topic and encompasses much more than painful menses, PCOS, and PMDD/PMS. But these are the conditions that I see the most, so I want to spend some time on them. I also will spend some time discussing vitamin D and insulin. I believe there is not an adequate amount of attention placed on these two hormones although they have a profound impact on brain function.

Painful Menses

Painful menses, known as dysmenorrhea, are very common. The menses may be regular or irregular with light or heavy menstrual flow. Menstrual pain can make a woman feel bad about herself and her womanhood. Her femaleness is hurting her. This can be very stressful for a woman, especially for the young. It is the young who suffer the most, with women between the ages of twenty and twenty-four having the most severe pain. Although there are many appropriate treatment modalities, only 15 percent of women will seek medical care for this condition. Painful periods are not normal and do not have to be endured.

Conventional medical management is either anti-inflammatory medication, such as ibuprofen, and/or birth control pills. Painful menses is the result of excess prostaglandins in the body. Prostaglandins constrict the blood vessels in the uterus and make the muscle layer contract, thus causing painful cramps. Therefore, the use of ibuprofen and other medications of that type are appropriate. Oral contraceptives are also a widely used treatment approach. The oral contraceptives will decrease the blood flow and may thereby lessen some of the discomfort.

Many women do not want to take birth control, or for some reason it is contraindicated. Some women cannot manage the anti-inflammatory medications due to their side effects (risk of GI bleed and others).

Lifestyle interventions and herbs are very helpful here. The lifestyle intervention begins with an anti-inflammatory diet. The anti-inflammatory diet consists of foods that are whole, unprocessed, and organic if possible. Avoiding dairy, gluten, and sugar reduces the inflammatory effect. Gastrointestinal complaints often accompany painful menses. Those complaints are often addressed with bitters (see below).

There are some supplements that are very helpful. Omega 3 fatty acids—EPA and DHA, which are found in fish oil—can be useful as an anti-inflammatory. Take a total of 3000 mg daily of the sum of these two fatty acids. The omega 3 fatty acids have been shown to reduce cramping by affecting the prostaglandin systems. The addition of calcium and magnesium together is very useful. The calcium seems to reduce cramping and irritability, and magnesium is a very safe muscle relaxant. Calcium is one of the most binding agents known, so using it in conjunction with magnesium is a good idea. If magnesium causes diarrhea, add calcium. If calcium causes constipation, add magnesium.

The herbal actions appropriate for the treatment of dysmenorrhea are anti-spasmodics, anti-inflammatories, and tonics.

The concept of a tonic is not present in the Western medical world. The idea of a tonic is that the herb nourishes the organ. Nourishing an organ means that it helps that organ thrive, build its cells, detoxify itself, and grow. A well-nourished organ will function optimally.

Herb	Herbal Action	How to Take/Use
Raspberry leaf tea	Uterine tonic, anti-spasmodic	Often sold as a tea in a tea bag. Place a tea bag in a cup and pour hot water over the bag and let sit for 10–15 minutes. Enjoy. Drink daily throughout the month for relief of menstrual cramps. May be consumed warm or cold. Traditional Medicinals makes a good quality tea.
Partridgeberry (Mitchella repens)	Uterine tonic, analgesic	As a tea, steep for 10–15 minutes and drink 1–3 cups daily. As a tincture (1:5) take 2–4 ml three times daily. As a crude herb (usually in capsule form) 1000–2000 mg daily. Hawaii pharm makes an alcohol-free extract. Take a dropper bulb four times daily.

Herb	Herbal Action	How to Take/Use
Black haw (*Viburnum prunofolium*)	Anti-inflammatory, β2 agonist	Simmer 1–2 teaspoons of bark in water for 10 minutes. Strain and drink 1 cup one to three times a day. Contains oxalic acid so do not use if there is a history of kidney stones.
Cramp bark (*Viburnum opulus*)	Anti-inflammatory, β2 agonist	Same as black haw but does not have oxalic acid so no concern for kidney stones.
Black cohosh (*Cimicifuga racemosa*)	Anti-inflammatory and anti-spasmodic, β2 agonist. Used historically for all problems with the uterus.	Take one Nature's Way green top 540 mg twice a day for three months, then one daily thereafter for maintenance.

A comment about bitters: bitters are just that, foods that have a bitter taste. The bitterness stimulates the bile and the liver to get digestion started. Often there are gastrointestinal complaints that accompany the painful menses. Irritable bowel syndrome is a common comorbidity. The effectiveness of the herbal treatment will be enhanced if the gut complaints are also addressed. Bitters can be purchased over the counter at liquor stores. Most contain alcohol, but Gallexier is one brand of bitters that is alcohol free. Organic Bitters is also an alcohol free bitter available at www.mercolamarket.com. Follow the directions on the product you purchase. Most often they are taken before the biggest meal/s of the day.

Premenstrual Syndrome (PMS)

One common complaint that I see as a psychiatrist is depression or moodiness prior to the menses. Premenstrual syndrome (PMS) is a real disorder. The changes in blood flow can be seen on SPECT scans. It's not uncommon to see a marked reduction of blood flow to the prefrontal cortex, with difficulty in attention, focus, and executive decision making only during the premenstrual time period.

Gynecologists often treat the mood component of PMS with oral birth control. Psychiatrists will treat the mood component by giving an increased dose of an anti-depressant prior to the menses. Both of these treatments can be helpful. But both of these approaches miss the underlying problem that causes the difficulty in the first place. There is an underlying hormonal dysregulation that occurs along with nutritional deficiencies, all of which can be addressed. Herbs can be very helpful for these circumstances.

The underlying hormonal dysregulation is a relative estrogen dominance—an increase in estrogen and a reduction of progesterone in the luteal phase (the later phase) of the menstrual cycle. With estrogen dominance comes an increase in norepinephrine, induced irritability and decreased progesterone, increased aldosterone with water retention, and increased prolactin with associated breast tenderness. Some women are very sensitive to prolactin increases. There is a decrease in endorphins, which leads to depression, sadness, and dysregulated hormones. There also is a decrease in dopamine. Dopamine is responsible for feeling good, having pleasure, enjoying activities, and also for focus and attention. For a summary of hormonal dysregulation, see the chart below.

The Hormonal Dysregulation in PMS Estrogen Dominance

Increased estrogen→Decreased progesterone

Increased norepinephrine→Increased irritability and decreased progesterone

Increased aldosterone→Increased water retention and bloating

Increased prolactin→Breast tenderness

Decrease in endorphins→Depression, sadness

Decrease in dopamine→Decrease in pleasure and enjoying activities and decrease in focus and attention

Nutrient deficiencies are a common underlying cause of the hormonal dysregulation in the first place. The nutrients B6, calcium, zinc, and magnesium are often low in PMS. There are many over-the-counter PMS supplement products that contain these nutrients. The form of B6 that is needed is an activated form called pyridoxal phosphate (p5p'). A B-complex is better than the B6 alone. Too much B6 may lead to paresthesias (pins and needles in the extremities) and may induce tremor of the limbs and/or torso and may be accompanied by an increase in anxiety. Also, since dopamine may be deficient there are some important mineral cofactors for the production of dopamine. Dopamine requires iron, zinc, and copper. All these nutrients are measurable in the blood. I highly recommend asking your doctor to measure them and I highly recommend measuring the magnesium as a red blood cell magnesium rather than a serum magnesium. The essential fatty acids and vitamin D should be supported as well.

There are different subtypes of PMS. I will go through each type and explain the herbal medicine that can be helpful for each.

PMS Anxious Type: The PMS Symptom Is Primarily One of Anxiety

Vitex (*Vitex agnus castus*) is also known as chasteberry or chaste tree. Vitex is known to reduce prolactin levels, increase progesterone levels (particularly in the last half of the cycle), and increase dopamine and endorphins. Nature's Way makes a good product of Vitex, 400 mg capsules, to be taken once daily. It will take three months to level out irregular menses and improve symptoms.

Nervines (also called nootropics) are also helpful. Nervines are herbs that support and nourish the nervous system. The herbs have their own special nuances and "personalities." Passionflower (*Passiflora incarnata*) is appropriate for those women who sacrifice themselves for others, such as family members. Lemon balm is perfect for the woman who is a busy bee, feeling out of sorts, and needs results now! Skullcap is perfect for that woman who becomes irritable and does not want to be touched ("Just leave me alone!"). Kava kava can also be used to reduce anxiety. I recommend taking kava as a tea in the afternoon. Yogi Tea makes a good product. If taken regularly, it is a good idea to have your doctor measure your liver enzymes as kava has been known to increase liver enzymes. All these herbs are available as a tea or an extract online and over the counter.

Adaptogens, herbs that help the body adapt to stress, are

also helpful here. Ashwagandha (*Withania somnifera*) is the most calming of the adaptogens. This adaptogen can be helpful for restful sleep. Follow the directions on the product that you purchase. Gaia Herbs makes a good product.

Eleuthero (*Eleutherococcus senticosus*), formerly known as Siberian ginseng, is helpful as well. This herb is particularly helpful for the young woman who is driven, works hard, plays hard, and hardly sleeps. Steep the herb for 20 minutes, strain, and drink. The whole herb tends to be slightly bitter, so I prefer to make it with almond milk and a bit of honey and cinnamon. It is quite nice.

Bitters can be an excellent addition to help the liver detoxify the body of the hormones. Bitters are herbs taken before the largest meal of the day and include Urban Moonshine (alcohol based), and Gallexier (alcohol free), among others.

PMS Carbohydrate Type: The PMS Symptom Is One Primarily of Carbohydrate Craving and Tension Headache

It is reasonable to crave carbohydrates prior to menstruation because the body uses carbohydrates to prepare itself for pregnancy. However, carbohydrate craving is very uncomfortable and a woman may feel she is not in control of her feelings, cravings, and behavior. There is a great deal of over-eating that is very uncomfortable and that makes the woman feel badly about herself. Devil's club is an herb that can help regulate the blood sugar and limit the carbohydrate cravings. It is available online as an alcohol-free tincture by Secrets of the Tribe. Follow the directions on the bottle of the product that you buy.

The first line treatment for PMS carbohydrate type is not an herb but a mineral: magnesium. Magnesium is enormously helpful and can be given before bed, which will also allow the woman to sleep a little better. The dose is 400–600 mg of magnesium citrate. If diarrhea develops, add calcium. The ratio of calcium to magnesium is 1:1. There are many over-the-counter preparations with a 1:1 ratio of magnesium to calcium. Another mineral, chromium, may be helpful as well in lessening carbohydrate cravings, although the research is mixed. The dose is 600–1000 mcg daily. There are many over-the-counter supplements available.

Diet is also very helpful here. A high protein, high fat, low carbohydrate diet is essential, but it is also hard to implement when there are strong cravings. Chromium is helpful for lowering the sugar craving, but a higher dose of around 1000 mg is needed. One tip is to open the capsule of chromium and place it directly on the tongue or place a bitter herb on the tongue. It will stop the craving for sweet and allow you to be able to follow the diet. Maintaining the high protein, high fat, and low carbohydrate diet throughout the month and not just prior to menses is also very helpful. The diet will help the body regulate the blood sugar and insulin levels.

Bitters are a must as well. The bitter flavor is a balance to the sweet flavor of the carbohydrate. Our drive for carbohydrates and sweets may partly be due to the fact that the typical American diet is low in bitter flavors. Bitter greens are being touted as health foods (which they are) and are finding their way onto grocery store shelves and into the salads purchased at restaurants. This is a good trend and I hope it continues. There are many bitter herbs that are applicable here: motherwort, dandelion root, gentian, and gymnema are common herbs available as extracts or tinctures. You can place a drop of the extract of gymnema on the tongue and it will block the taste of sweet. Bitters should be taken before the largest meal of the day. An alcohol-based preparation is Urban Moonshine, or an alcohol-free preparation is Gallexier or Organic Bitters from www.mercolamarket.com.

Adaptogens are non-toxic herbs that help the body manage stress. There are several with the ability to modulate blood sugar: Devils club (*Oplopanax horridus*), eleuthero (*Eleutherococcus senticosus*), and panax ginseng. Cinnamon is also a great blood sugar reducer. Simply adding cinnamon to your everyday foods can improve your fasting blood sugar. You can add ground cinnamon to yogurt or put a cinnamon stick in coffee as it is brewing or dripping for added flavor and blood sugar reduction.

PMS-Depression Type: The Primary Symptom Is Depression

The technical definition is that the depression only occurs during the week prior to menses, but with a careful history taking you will often find there is an underlying dysthymia (a mild depressed mood that does not meet criteria for major depression but is chronic) throughout the month. This sets the stage for depression during the PMS time.

One very useful herb is Black cohosh (*Actea racemosa*). Black cohosh, 540 mg two to four times per day, acts like a selective serotonin reuptake inhibitor (SSRI). This increases serotonin for mood enhancement. The use of 5-htp, the precursor to serotonin, is helpful for sleep and mood enhancement as well. You can go up on the doses of 5-htp to 300 mg at bedtime if needed. The body also needs an adequate amount of B6, particularly the p5p' activated version. Again, the whole B complex is safer and a good way to avoid the toxicity of excess B6.

St. John's wort can be helpful as well, especially when taken with vitex. Vitex is helpful for the physical symptoms but not the depressive ones. St. John's wort can improve the mood and is very relaxing. St. John's wort interacts with medication by inducing the P450 enzyme system and will reduce the amount of certain medications in the bloodstream. Be sure to check with your health care provider if you are taking any prescribed medications.

Depression is often accompanied by anxiety and brain fog. Passionflower (*Passiflora*) is an excellent herb to improve the anxiety; bacopa (*Bacopa monnieri*) is an anti-anxiety herb that also helps with brain fog, and Rhodiola (*Rhodiola rosea*) is an excellent adaptogen that helps with physical and mental fatigue.

PMS-Hyperhydration Type: The Primary Symptom for This Type Is Swelling

The swelling can be quite uncomfortable with accompanying breast tenderness. Increasing magnesium is helpful. Ginkgo biloba is helpful for improving fluid movement through the vasculature, reducing breast tenderness and leg swelling. There are a few herbs that are helpful as mild diuretics: dandelion root (*Taraxacum officianale*), nettleleaf (*Urtica dioica*), and skullcap (*Scutalleria lateriflora*) tea. These herbs are high in potassium and help excrete sodium and water. These herbs are readily available as commercial teas.

PMS-Painful Type: The Primary Symptom for This Type Is Pain

It is an awful feeling to have pain before the menses and to feel that your body is hurting you. Vitex (*Vitex agnus castus*) increases endogenous opioids and can be quite helpful here. There are different types of pain and specific herbs address the specific type of pain.

Some women experience tension headaches prior to their menses. Wood betony, *Stachys officianalis,* is an excellent herb for relieving pain in the muscles of the head, neck, and shoulders. Wood betony is available from herb websites, www.mountainroseherbs.com or www.starwest-botanicals.com. Make as a tea and drink 3–4 cups daily or purchase as an extract or tincture. An alcohol-free liquid extract is sold by www.hawaiipharm.com. Follow the directions on the bottle and use freely the week prior to menses.

Below is a chart of pain-relieving herbs for PMS:

Type of Pain	Matching Herb
Dull, achy pain	Black cohosh (*Actea racemosa*)
Tense, spasmodic pain	Cramp bark (*Viburnum opulus*)
Fibromyalgia pain	Rhodiola (*Rhodiola rosea*)
Tight and tense	Valerian root (*Valeriana officinalis*)
Tension headache	Wood betony (*Stachys officinalis*)
Pelvic pain, cramps	Partridge berry (*Mitchella repens*)
Menstrual cramps and low back pain	Black haw (*Viburnum prunifolium*)
Anti-spasmodic, uterine tonic	Raspberry leaf tea (*Rubus idaeus*)

Work with your health care provider to establish the best treatment for you.

8

POLYCYSTIC OVARY SYNDROME (PCOS)

Polycystic ovary syndrome (PCOS) is a common problem for women. Approximately 21 percent of women are diagnosed with the condition and unfortunately the number of cases is rising. Two-thirds of infertile women will have PCOS. The syndrome causes a great deal of distress for women and is a significant threat to health. The symptoms of PCOS include evidence of hyperandrogenism, such as facial hair and adult acne. There is a strong association with obesity and insulin resistance. This is why I find it distressing when dermatology treats adult acne without an investigation into insulin resistance or hormonal irregularities. The cost to health is very high. PCOS is too often undiagnosed. Perhaps this is because the name of the syndrome is misleading and there is no agreement on the diagnostic criteria.

According to an independent panel convened by the National Institutes of Health the problem is that the name of the condition focuses on a criterion—ovarian cysts—but the presence of cysts is not necessary or sufficient to diagnose the syndrome. In 2013, the panel recommended assigning a new name that more accurately reflects the disorder,[9] but as of this writing the syndrome has not yet been renamed. It is important to note that it is possible to have the PCOS syndrome *without* ovarian cysts being present.

The diagnosis of PCOS is defined differently depending on which professional society you consult.[10] The Rotterdam diagnosis criteria is two out of three of the following:

1. Anovulation (absence of ovulation) or oligo-ovulation (lessened ovulation)

2. Hyperandrogenism (elevated testosterone on blood testing)

3. Polycystic ovaries on ultrasound

The Androgen Excess and PCOS Society has a similar definition:

1. Hyperandrogenism (clinical or biochemical excess testosterone shown on blood tests)

2. Ovarian dysfunction as evidenced by oligo-anovulation and/or polycystic ovaries

3. Exclusion of other related disorders

What is clear is that the presence of ovarian dysfunction is necessary, but the presence of ovarian cysts is not necessary. The presence of androgenism, either clinically present (adult-onset acne) or found on bloodwork is key.

The health risks to the woman include obesity and insulin resistance. The obesity is mostly found around the waist, which is a characteristic of metabolic syndrome. These two conditions, obesity and insulin resistance, lead to an increased risk of type 2 diabetes, estrogen dominance with associated dysfunctional uterine bleeding, increased risk of heart disease, increased risk of breast cancer, and increased risk of uterine cancer. Most women with this syndrome are not able to conceive.

Lifestyle interventions can be helpful for PCOS, beginning with a low carbohydrate diet such as the Paleo diet. For those unfamiliar with the Paleo diet, it is a diet based on ancestral eating prior to the development of agriculture, so no grains or legumes are consumed. The diet consists of eating meat (if it walks, swims, or flies it is free game), eating vegetables and fruits that can be gathered (anything that grows above ground). There is also no dairy. The Paleo diet is a low carbohydrate diet that can improve insulin levels and reduce blood sugar.

Exercise is also key. Exercise is well known to reduce insulin levels and improve sensitivity of the cells to insulin.

There are some herbs and supplements that can be helpful to improve the syndrome.

Herbs for PCOS

Herb	Herbal Action
Cinnamon (true and false cinnamon)	3 g/day (a little more than a teaspoon) decreases blood sugar; can also take as the essential oil in a capsule
Triphala (*Amla*)	2–3 g/day improves insulin sensitivity, good for the cardiovascular and GI systems
Spearmint tea (*Mentha spicata*)	2 cups of tea daily. Decreases testosterone and increases SHBG (the metabolic bus that carries hormones around in the serum and is low in PCOS)

| Modified TJ-68 Shakuyaku-kanzo-to, Chinese herbal remedy with white Peonia (*Peony alactoflora*) and Licorice (*Glycyrrhiza glabra*) | The original preparation is equal parts of the peonia and the licorice. Due to the ability of licorice to raise blood pressure, Dr. Low Dog recommends 2 parts peonia, 1 part licorice. The effects of these two are additive; licorice and peonia decrease androgens and peonia decreases insulin and blood sugar. This has to be mixed for you by an herbalist. |

Do *not* use vitex in PCOS because it will worsen the situation.

Supplements for PCOS

Supplement	Dosages
Magnesium	600 mg daily
Chromium	1000 mg daily
N-acetyl cysteine (NAC)	1200 mg daily, improves detox
Alpha lipoic acid	600 mg twice a day
Myo-inositol	4 grams daily improves metabolic syndrome[11] and mimics insulin function
D-chiro inositol	1 gram daily decreases androgens[12]

Important Note: If you think you may have PCOS, please work with your health care provider. It is a complicated syndrome with far reaching consequences. It is important that you are followed and monitored by a health care provider.

9

THE VITAMIN D CONNECTION

Vitamin D is the forgotten vitamin. It is critical to many normal biological processes and is necessary for health, and in the past was rarely measured by doctors. For years, I have routinely ordered vitamin D levels in my psychiatric patients. I am happy to see that measuring the vitamin D level is now becoming more common with general practitioners in their annual physical workups, and checking for low vitamin D levels is slowly becoming a mainstream medical practice.

But why is a vitamin included in a section on hormones? The reason is that vitamin D is both a hormone and a vitamin. It is a vitamin in that we can consume it in our food as ergocalciferol (vitamin D2). It is a hormone because it is made in one part of the body, secreted into the bloodstream, and has an action on another part of the body (the definition of a hormone). It is called a seco-steroid hormone and is one of the most potent steroids in the body.

There is a lot of research on vitamin D.[13] As I've said, vitamin D is critical to health. There are vitamin D receptors in all the organs of the body, and vitamin D has influence on the heart, the blood vessels, the bones, the muscles, the immune system, and the brain. It is a support for immune function, so an adequate vitamin D level is needed to fight infection.

Vitamin D is well known to be necessary for the formation of strong bones and to prevent osteoporosis and fractures. What is less well known about vitamin D is its importance in other systems of the body. It is necessary for strong muscles, not just bones, and will reduce the risk of falls in elders. Vitamin D reduces the risk of cancer, improves cancer survivability, reduces heart disease, is necessary for our absorption of calcium and phosphorus, and improves mood. Vitamin D is also key for cognitive function. Patients with Alzheimer's disease often have low vitamin D; those with mild cognitive impairment, likewise have low vitamin D. Given that Alzheimer's disease is reaching epidemic proportions and affecting more women than men, it is important to utilize all the tools that we have to prevent and treat cognitive impairment. Vitamin D is an inexpensive and easy way to accomplish that.

The blood test that should be ordered is 25 OH vitamin D. The level that is most efficacious in the serum is 60–80 ng/ml (156 nmol/l to 208 nmol/l). I have personally treated some very deep bipolar depression episodes by elevating vitamin D to the 60 ng/ml level with very good success.

Since vitamin D has far reaching effects on the body, it is an easy and inexpensive way to improve health. Vitamin D levels should be tested regularly. Since we do make vitamin D from exposure to the sun, I often measure the vitamin D level in the late fall—October or November. You want to maintain an adequate level of vitamin D in the serum throughout the winter months to maintain mood and prevent the winter blues.

Summary of Some Key Effects of Vitamin D

Organ system	Effects
Mental health	Improves mood, reduces depression, and prevents the winter blues
Brain	Improves cognition, prevents mild cognitive impairment and Alzheimer's disease
Heart	Improves endothelial function of the blood vessel, cardiac function, improves hypertension
Cancer	By regulating cell growth, it reduces risk of and improves survival from numerous cancers including, breast, colon, and lymphoma
Bone health	Prevents fracture and osteoporosis, partly due to the increased ability to absorb and utilize calcium
Muscle health	An under-appreciated benefit of vitamin D is that it reduces sarcopenia and muscle weakness in elders leading to fall prevention
Immune health	Vitamin D reduces infection and stimulates the immune system's ability to recover from infection
Diabetes	Improves blood sugar and insulin function
Autoimmune diseases	Due to the improvement of immune function autoimmune diseases are less frequent

Vitamin D is an anti-inflammatory and improves endothelial function with reduction of MI risk.

10

THE INSULIN CONNECTION

Insulin is a hormone most well-known for the regulation of blood sugar. Insulin is responsible for moving blood sugar out of the serum and into the muscles during exercise to provide a source of energy. The most well-known medical condition that involves insulin is diabetes. Diabetes type 1 results from an autoimmune process that damages the pancreas and therefore the body is not able to manufacture insulin in sufficient quantity to utilize blood sugar as fuel. Diabetes type 2 results when the blood sugar is chronically elevated and the body becomes resistant to the effects of the insulin when it is present in adequate amounts. This condition is known as insulin resistance. The consequence of insulin resistance involves a marked dysregulation of fat metabolism. Part of the job of insulin is to move the glucose into the muscle cells for energy and the rest goes into storage as fat cells. Fat cells are themselves metabolically active.

Why would you want your psychiatrist to be concerned about insulin? What does it have to do with depression?

Over my years of practice, one of the things that I have observed over and over again is that high blood glucose levels, insulin resistance, depressed mood, and poor eating habits all seem to appear together. I began measuring fasting insulin on a regular basis, and I consistently find that an elevated reading is associated with emotional dysregulation and dysfunctional eating. Leptin and ghrelin (the hormone of satiety) are more directly related to the sensation of satiety, but insulin seems to correlate with emotional distress and often carbohydrate craving. I have no proof, but I often wonder if insulin becomes elevated as a reaction to inflammation.

What I have learned from this is that an elevated insulin level with the associated insulin resistance is a marker of the metabolic effect of stress, leading to inflammation, cognitive impairment, and emotional dysregulation. Elevated insulin is a consequence, I believe, not a cause. I am not alone in these observations.

Alzheimer's disease, growing at epidemic proportions, is sometimes referred to as type 3 diabetes. Dr. Dale Bredesen,[14] the author of *The End of Alzheimer's*, has this to say:

> This insulin resistance contributes not only to type 2 diabetes, fatty liver, and metabolic syndrome, but also to Alzheimer's disease. The reason: *Insulin signaling is one of the most important signals for the support of neuron survival.* Insulin binds to the insulin receptor and triggers signaling that supports neuronal survival; this survival signal is blunted by chronically high insulin levels. But that's not the only connection between chronically high insulin levels and Alzheimer's. (Emphasis mine)

Think about this not just for Alzheimer's disease but for the garden variety depression. How can you expect the brain to function well, to be happy, have good relationships with others, and feel good about yourself when the neurons are fighting for their very survival? A chief complaint of depressed mood is brain fog and difficulty with concentration. It's no wonder there is brain fog if one of the underlying mechanisms is a neuronal fight for survival.

The next point that Dr. Bredesen makes is that the same enzyme is used to remove Amyloid plaque (found in Alzheimer's disease) as is used to remove insulin once it has done its job—insulin-degrading enzyme (IDE). If the IDE is busy removing excess insulin it is less available for removing Amyloid plaque.

Insulin has other interactions as well. Increased insulin decreases sex-hormone binding globulin (SHBG). The SHBG is the bus that carries the sex hormones around in the blood-stream. When there is less SHBG, there are more hormones in the bloodstream, but they are unregulated. This can lead to estrogen dominance in women, leading to emotional dysregulation secondary to hormonal dysregulation. (See the information on PMS in chapter 7.)

There may be many other interactions found in future research, but the relationship between elevated insulin levels, high level of anxiety, depressed mood, and poor dietary habits that are high glycemic in nature is consistently present.

There are many natural approaches to lowering blood sugar and insulin levels. The first one is not an herb, but a mineral: magnesium. Taking an adequate amount of magnesium can be useful in this regard. An adequate dose will vary person to person, but 400–600 mg of magnesium nightly is a good place to start. An excess of magnesium can lead to diarrhea so it may have to be balanced by calcium. Also, the form of magnesium L-threonate may be better tolerated and better absorbed without the GI distress. The L-threonate form readily passes the blood brain barrier. The dose for magnesium L-threonate is 2000 mg daily.

Cinnamon will lower blood sugar and insulin levels readily. You can add cinnamon, a sweet herb, into your diet easily. Put a cinnamon stick in coffee as it is being brewed or add cinnamon to a smoothie. You need about a teaspoon of cinnamon daily for a therapeutic effect.

Berberine, the active ingredient in Oregon grape root, Golden Seal, Coptis, and others is an excellent way to lower blood sugar and insulin levels. Berberine does interact with the cytochrome P450 (CYP 450) pathway in the liver. Specifically, berberine inhibits the enzymes 2D6, 3A4, and 2C9. If you are taking a medication that is metabolized by one of these enzymes, the level of that medication may rise in your bloodstream. This does not mean you cannot take the medication and the berberine together, but it may mean that as long as you are taking the berberine you may need to lower the dose of the medication to maintain the appropriate serum level. Berberine has a short half-life, so 500 mg three times a day is recommended.

Bitter melon (*Momordica charantia*) is a fruit that, as its name implies, is bitter. It is consumed as a food in Africa and Asia and somewhat resembles a cucumber. It is used for its bitter quality to balance the flavor of food. It has been used as a traditional remedy for elevated blood sugar for centuries. The food has a more bitter taste than is agreeable to the Western palate, so most people consume it as a capsule, although it is sometimes put in smoothies. The dose also varies. If you are taking it to lower blood sugar, be sure you monitor your blood sugar. The dose is 500 mg to 1500 mg daily depending on the needs of the person. It may also lower blood pressure so if you have high blood pressure, be sure to monitor your pressure.

Gymnema sylvestre, also known as gumar, is well studied for the reduction of blood glucose and the reduction of type 2 diabetes. Many type 2 diabetics are able to stop their medication after taking this herb and improving their diet. One way that *Gymnema sylvestre* works is by reducing the craving for sugary foods, although the clinical results are variable. It may also inhibit the absorption of sugar in the small intestine.[15] The dose is 500 mg of the extract standardized to 25 percent *Gymnemic* acid before the main meal of the day. Do not take on an empty stomach or if pregnant.

There are many culinary herbs that are helpful for blood sugar control as well. These include marjoram, oregano, sage, rosemary, and cloves, and of course, my favorite listed above, cinnamon. Simply adding these herbs to your food will bring you great delight in culinary flavors and also yield medicinal benefits.

Summary Table of Herbs and Spices That Lower Blood Sugar

Cinnamon	1 teaspoon daily, use as a flavoring in food, coffee, smoothies.
Magnesium L-threonate	2000 mg of magnesium L-threonate. Many companies offer this product but 3–4 capsules daily are needed.

Bitter melon (*Momordica charantia*)	500 mg to 1500 mg daily depending on the amount of blood sugar lowering that is needed. Since this is a very bitter herb it may be more agreeable as a capsule. Monitor your blood sugar and blood pressure if taking this herb and you have diabetes and hypertension.
Gumar (*Gymnema sylvestre*)	Take 500 mg extract before the largest meal of the day. This reduces the craving for sweet and may inhibit sugar absorption from the small intestine. Do not take on an empty stomach or if pregnant.
Culinary herbs: marjoram, oregano, sage, rosemary, cinnamon, and cloves	Incorporate these herbs into your diet. Eat them freely.

11

OTHER TREATMENTS FOR DEPRESSION

In this chapter, I would like to explore other popular and effective treatments for depression.

Psychotherapy

Let's leave the realm of physiology and move into the realm of the psyche for a moment. Let's talk about psychotherapy.

Psychotherapy is often the cornerstone of treatment for depression (and anxiety). Deep-seated feelings of anger, disappointment, and fear of one's own emotions are all important issues to work through in therapy. I remember a young man who suffered from deep depression. He smoked marijuana daily to avoid feeling the deep-seated despair he had buried. I could see that despair in him, and he acknowledged that it was there. When I told him that he had to work through that despair to resolve his depression, he refused. He wanted to fix his feelings of depression some other way. But there is no other way; those buried feelings (whatever they were) were the wellspring of his depression. Without exploring them in a safe environment and helping him express and resolve them, they would always torture him. Marijuana and medications and natural remedies would not matter. He was not open to my perception, and needless to say he did not pursue therapy. I have not had contact with him since that initial visit, but I still worry about his well-being.

A case like this makes me sad. It is scary for someone to face up to their feelings, especially when those feelings are strong. Some people are more sensitive to their feelings than others, and the idea of exploring strong emotions is just too overwhelming for them. This was the case, in my opinion, with the young man mentioned above. I also suspect this is one reason medications fail. Medications cannot cure the deep-seated anguish of a person's life, and neither can herbs or supplements. But therapy, when properly done, can make a big difference. Medications, herbs, and supplements *can* help buffer some of the intensity of those feelings, making it possible to work through them in therapy. In this manner therapy and medication, both pharmaceutical and nutraceutical, can work well together.

Cognitive Behavioral Therapy and Eye Movement Desensitization and Reprocessing

Cognitive behavioral therapy (CBT) has been the most well studied as a treatment for depression. Most of the research shows that CBT and medication work better together than either one alone.[16] Research also shows that the addition of therapy helps maintain the gains made even after medication has been discontinued, a claim that cannot be made by medication treatment alone.[17]

Cognitive behavioral therapy is based on the idea that your thinking determines your feelings and that by reframing how you think about things you can change your feelings about yourself and your life's situation. CBT focuses on the automatic negative thoughts (Dr. Amen calls these ANTs) we have about ourselves and teaches people to reframe them, thereby changing their feelings. The *New Oxford Textbook of Psychiatry*, 2012, lists the following as some examples of ANTs:

- ***Black-and-white*** (also called all-or-nothing): Situations are seen as an either/or scenario. Example: "If I don't take first prize, I'm a complete failure."

- ***Fortune-telling*** (also called catastrophizing): This is when the future is predicted to be negative, ignoring other possible, more likely outcomes. Example: "I'm going to say the wrong thing and she'll never talk to me again."

- ***Disqualifying or discounting the positive:*** Positive qualities, outcomes, or actions don't count. Example: "I won the race, but it was just beginner's luck. I'm not that fast."

- ***Emotional reasoning:*** Thinking something must be true because you "feel" (actually believes) it so strongly, despite evidence to the contrary. Example: "Sure, I got a high grade on the test, but I still feel like an idiot."

- ***Labeling:*** Putting a fixed label on oneself or others, discounting any evidence that might lead to a more favorable conclusion. Example: "I'm a loser. I will never be good enough."

- ***Magnification/minimization:*** Judging oneself, another person, or a situation, focusing on the negative and/or ignoring the positive. Example: "Making that mistake shows how incompetent I am. Getting that promotion doesn't mean I deserve it."

- **Selective abstraction** (also called mental filter): Paying undue attention to one negative detail instead of seeing the whole picture. Example: "Getting a C in chemistry proves I'm a terrible student [even though I got A's in every other subject]."

- **Mind reading:** Believing that you know what others are thinking, and assuming they think the worst. Example: "My boss gave me this assignment because he thinks I can't handle anything more challenging."

- **Overgeneralization:** Making a negative conclusion that goes far beyond the current situation. Example: "Because I was tongue-tied when he caught me off guard, proves that I will never be a good public speaker."

- **Personalization:** Believing that you are the reason for other people behaving negatively. Example: "My boss didn't say good morning to me because he hates me."

- **Imperatives** (also called "should" and "must" statements): Having a fixed idea of how you or others should behave, and you exaggerate how bad it is that these expectations are not met. Example: "I should have submitted that report earlier. I'm going to get fired."

- ***Tunnel vision:*** You only see the negative aspect of a situation. Example: "I can't believe the restaurant we wanted to go to is closed. I know we have a reservation at the new place just down the street, but our plans fell apart."

If you watch yourself over the course of a day, you may find yourself saying similar things to yourself. It is fascinating how often these negative thoughts come to us and how often we criticize ourselves for simple life events.

I will often recommend CBT along with all the lifestyle interventions discussed so far. To my knowledge, the research that has been done on CBT has been with medication. It would be an interesting research project to evaluate CBT along with medication and the herbal and lifestyle recommendations made in this book. I believe you would have a better outcome and one that was longer lasting.

Another style of therapy I will recommend is eye movement desensitization and reprocessing (EMDR). EMDR was developed specifically for a particular trauma and is used to treat post-traumatic stress disorder (PTSD). When a person experiences a traumatic event, the brain acknowledges that traumatic event. The person has an emotional reaction to that event and the brain then builds a bridge between them. The job of the EMDR therapist is to get the patient to re-experience the trauma, complete with the emotions and kinesthetic sensations (such as smell, taste, sounds), and then the therapist moves the eyes or makes a sound to break the bridge. This style of therapy has documented efficacy for post-traumatic stress disorder.[18]

Physical Therapeutic Approaches

Neurofeedback

Neurofeedback—a subset of biofeedback—is also called (electro-encephalograph) EEG biofeedback. The patient is given a computerized EEG to develop a map of the electrical waves of the brain. The brain is then stimulated through the visual system to balance the firing; it quiets those brain waves that are overly active and stimulates those waves that are not active enough.

Neurofeedback is helpful for the treatment of attention deficit disorder, major depression, generalized anxiety, and brain injury. A common disorder that I see in clinic is brain injury from concussion. Sometimes the concussion is from playing football in school, sometimes it is from accidents, but whatever the cause the concussion leaves a lasting impression on the brain. Along with other treatments (hyperbaric oxygen therapy, supplementation, etc.), neurofeedback is a must for brain repair. Neurofeedback improves the processing speed of the brain which is often lessened because of injury.

Alpha Stim

The alpha stim is an FDA approved medical device that clips to the earlobes. It is indicated for the treatment of anxiety, depression, insomnia, and chronic pain. Some patients find benefit from wearing it. It is effective in as little as twenty minutes and can be worn at home. It does not require going anywhere, seeing a therapist, or any additional cost.[19]

Interactive Metronome/Cerebellar Enhancement

Interactive metronome is an evidence-based computer program designed to improve attention, focus, emotional regulation, cognition, and coordination in children and adults. It is helpful for children with learning disabilities, adults with early stages of dementia, obsessive compulsive disorder, and those who have attention deficit disorder of all ages. This technique is extremely well-researched and one I recommend regularly. The interactive metronome website has a long bibliography of research papers. For more information I recommend their site, www.interactivemetronome.com.[20] The research bibliography can be found here: www.interactivemetronome.com/images/pdfs/IM-RESEARCH-BIBLIOGRAPHY.pdf.

Hyperbaric Oxygen Therapy

With head trauma such as concussion and traumatic brain injury, my first treatment modality recommendation is hyperbaric oxygen therapy. Dr. Daniel Amen has done a lot of the research on the use of the hyperbaric oxygen therapy after football injuries because of his work with the National Football League. Now, sometimes you can see the hyperbaric chambers on the sidelines of the football games.[21] There are not a lot of studies on the use of hyperbaric oxygen therapy for the treatment of brain injury, but there are many practitioners using the technique with good success.

Clinically, I find that some cases of treatment resistant depression are associated with brain trauma and injury. Consider this gentleman, Edward, who came to the clinic complaining of depression, difficulty thinking like he was developing dementia, trouble with focus, and no response to treatment. His brain scan is shown below.

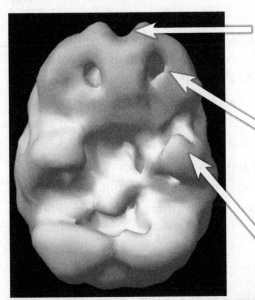

Note the reduced function of the frontal lobe, associated with difficulty in decision making

Note the marked reduction of prefrontal function associated with focus and concentration difficulty

Note the marked reduction in size of the temporal lobes, associated with memory deficits

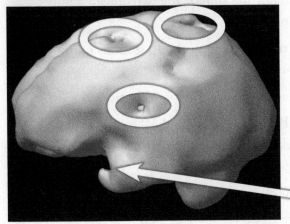

Note the irregularity of the parietal lobe and the small hole on the side and the two holes on the top. The parietal lobes help with navigation and attention.

Note the small temporal lobe.

Figure 11.1 This is a forty-year-old gentleman, Edward, who became depressed five years ago and has not responded to treatment. His scans show common signs of physical injury that we see at the Amen clinic. *Used with permission.*

After a brain injury, the brain may lose the reserve to biochemically respond to medical treatment. The way the scan pictures are made is by using a tracer material that is injected into the bloodstream, which attaches to the red blood cells and will go wherever red blood cells travel. When there is a decrease in function of the lobe, the lobe will pick up less tracer material which will show on the scan picture as a deficit or as a hole. A decrease in tracer material to an area is representative of a decrease in function of that lobe and shows up as a deficit or a hole. Edward did not have the brain reserve to respond to appropriate treatment and is suffering as a result.

What follows is a list of treatment recommendations that I made for Edward.

For brain injury

- 3000 mg daily of the sum of the two omega 3 fatty acids EPA and DHA.

- Hyperbaric oxygen therapy, for 40 sessions minimum, at an ATA of 1.3 to 2.0.

- Neurofeedback twice weekly for 20 sessions.

- Dr. Amen's BrainMD Brain and Memory Power Boost—an excellent supplement of nutrients designed specifically for brain repair.

- Myer's Cocktail, an IV of magnesium and B vitamins for nutritional support for his cortisol-stress system as I suspected he was depleted and has a melancholic depression described earlier.

Nutritional support for depression

- SAMe, beginning at 400 mg daily. I recommended this to improve the mood and to help stimulate the brain.

For the complaints of lack of focus

- I recommended the interactive metronome.

To improve sleep

- He had trouble staying asleep, so I recommended L-tryptophan 500 mg for a week, working up to 1500 mg if needed.

For diet

- I recommended the paleo (no grains, low carbohydrate, no dairy) diet with a focus on high fiber vegetables. The keto diet is the one that has been most studied to repair the brain, but it was too much of a change from his daily eating style.

Exercise

- I recommended he try and get aerobic exercise 20 minutes at a time three times a week.

For stress reduction

- I recommended mindfulness meditation and the Inner Balance app, a biofeedback app by Heart Math.

Herbal recommendations

- *Bacopa monnieri* 600 mg daily for brain function and to reduce brain fog. This is a complement to the nutrients in Brain and Memory Power Boost.

- Lion's mane is an excellent mushroom extract to support the underlying energy and immune system that in Edward was so depleted.

Medication

- I started Edward on desvenlafaxine 25 mg. This is a low dose, but I always start low and go slow to avoid side effects.

This case is an excellent example of how to use all the tools we have at our disposal together. I have every expectation that Edward will make great progress if he can implement these recommendations. It is possible that he will begin to feel better right away, but it will take three months for the brain to begin to heal and all the nutritional and herbal recommendations to have a full effect.

PART III

HERBAL MEDICINE FOR ANXIETY

• • • • • • • • • • • • • • • •

12

ANXIETY DISORDERS AND TREATMENTS

Anxiety is a normal human emotion that we all experience. Common scenarios are anxiety before a big exam, anxiety before a date, anxiety before a job interview, worrying about money, being afraid of social interactions. What exactly is it that we are experiencing? Why do we have anxiety?

Anxiety is important for us because it helps us identify a threat or a danger. All of the situations above are examples of worry about the future and things one cannot control. If we are uncertain about the outcome, we often experience fear, worry, and anxiety.

Anxiety is processed through the amygdala in the brain. If you are out for a walk and you hear footsteps behind you, your brain will register that and you will have to decide if the footsteps are a danger. Is it a stranger following you? Is it your spouse? Or possibly your child? All of those possible scenarios are registered by the amygdala to discern danger. We need anxiety. Those footsteps may be harmless, but the amygdala helps us determine if our safety is compromised.

The amygdala is an almond-shaped organ in the temporal lobe, close to the hippocampus (the memory center). It has

115

many connections with the rest of the brain. The amygdala interacts with the hypothalamus (the endocrine system), the thalamus (an emotional center), the hippocampus (the memory center), the brainstem (for motor action), the orbital prefrontal cortex (associated with focus and concentration), and the anterior cingulate cortex (associated with obsessions). The important component of these connections is that they are reciprocal, meaning a two-way street.

What is significant about these connections is that the amygdala has connections throughout the brain with broad reaching effects. If the amygdala interprets the footsteps as a danger, your endocrine system is turned on through the hypothalamus and cortisol can be activated along with the sympathetic nervous system, preparing you for fight or flight. The thalamus can trigger strong emotions and you may not be able to think clearly; the hippocampus is triggered, and you may or may not remember what happened. This process is critical to our survival. It is a normal process. However, it can become a chronic process. When chronic, it is similar to the stress reaction described in chapter 5, "The Cortisol Connection."

Like stress, when the anxiety is acute and short-lived it is a normal response to a life experience. However, like stress, when it becomes chronic, long-standing, and detached from the emotional underpinnings, it becomes a disorder. Anxiety disorders, especially panic disorder, often come "out of the blue." There is no conscious awareness of the cause or the emotional trigger. This disconnection is one of the more frightening aspects of anxiety disorders.

Anxiety is miserable; everyone hates the feeling. Depression and anxiety are often found together. Sometimes the brain will shut down and become depressed, just because the feeling of anxiety is so awful. Anxiety has two flavors: worry and fear. Both worry and fear are present in the anxious person, but often one will predominate. Sometimes, when I ask the person, they say the two feelings are equal. Whatever the balance, they are almost always present together.

There are five anxiety disorders identified by the DSM-5; all of them involve the combination of fear and worry. They are:

1. Generalized anxiety disorder

2. Panic disorder

3. Social anxiety disorder

4. Post-traumatic stress disorder

5. Obsessive-compulsive disorder

Anxiety disorders are the most prevalent of the mental health disorders and are more common in women. Anxiety as a disorder usually begins in the preteen and teen years; the mean age of onset of anxiety disorders is age eleven.[22] Many people will suffer throughout their lives and not seek professional help. This may be, in part, because they are afraid of leaving their homes, afraid of being judged, and in my experience, often they are afraid of treatment. In my clinical experience they also are very sensitive to side effects from medication, and I speculate that they have difficulty with detoxification.

Psychologically, there are well-known triggers for the feeling of anxiety. These triggers are:

- Loss of relationship, real or perceived
- Loss of control
- Anger that cannot be safely expressed

The loss of relationship can be the feeling that your significant other will leave you (perceived loss) or that your significant other packed up and moved out (real loss). Loss of control is a common, everyday experience for most. We cannot control the stock market, the weather, the actions of other people, things that happen, or what will happen. We cannot control if we get a job or a raise or anything else that we are looking forward to. One of the most difficult things we cannot control is the behavior of other people. Children and spouses can be especially difficult in this regard because we love them and want the best for them. One cannot control the drug addiction behavior of a child or a spouse for example. This can be very anxiety producing. Suppressed anger may also cause anxiety. Sometimes, anger may not be able to be safely expressed. The boss has insulted you once again and it makes you angry, but if you tell him off you will be fired. If these life experiences occur when there is chronic, underlying stress you may experience unbearable anxiety or a panic attack.

Anxiety, as described above, is mediated through the hypothalamic-pituitary-adrenal (HPA) axis. The stressor is perceived by the amygdala, which triggers the sympathetic nervous system to release norepinephrine and the HPA axis to release cortisol. The sympathetic nervous system is the "fight or flight" system of neurotransmitters that allow us to respond to a stressor by either fighting or running away. The neurotransmitter that is associated with the sympathetic nervous system is norepinephrine and its precursor, dopamine. It gives us energy, alertness, and mobilizes blood sugar to the muscles so we can use them rapidly. Norepinephrine is the neurotransmitter that makes us feel agitated; it raises our blood pressure. In response to the increase in norepinephrine, the HPA axis releases cortico-releasing hormone so our adrenal gland can release cortisol and we have the hormonal support to address and manage the stressor.

The brain likes balance, so it makes a neurotransmitter to calm everything down, too. That neurotransmitter is gamma-aminobutyric acid (GABA). It is made from the amino acid glutamate and is found in numerous interneurons (neurons that connect two other neurons together). GABA has an inhibitory effect on the brain. GABA is what calms us down, slows the breathing, decreases the blood sugar, and slows the heart rate. GABA has a profound effect on the feeling of anxiety, and it is from studying the effect of GABA that we have been able to understand anxiety.

The neurological pathways from the amygdala to other areas of the brain that occur with anxiety are also the neurological pathways that are active in major depression. Those pathways are influenced by serotonin and therefore serotonin enhancing agents, such as anti-depressant medications, improve anxiety as well. This overlap also explains the close relationship between anxiety and depression.

The physiology of anxiety as outlined above has been my understanding since I completed my psychiatric residency. However, new research is broadening the understanding of how people feel anxious and opening up the opportunity for new approaches to treatment. Opioid and adenosine receptors are being examined for their effect on the experience of anxiety. Both of these receptors are influenced by herbs that have been used historically for the management of the anxious state.

The nature of herbal medicine is that the herb itself is complex and has complex actions, which means it binds to multiple receptor sites. As we review the herbs most commonly used to calm anxiety, you will see that the herbs have more than one action and that there is not a specific herb for a specific anxiety disorder. The biggest difference that I see between conventional psychiatry and herbal medicine is the target of the remedy. In psychopharmacology the target is the receptor site of the neurotransmitters, but there is no interest in the connection with cortisol or an attempt to modulate the cortisol response. In herbal medicine, the emphasis is on the cortisol response and its effect on the neurotransmitter functions but not a specific receptor site. See chapter 5, "The Cortisol Connection," for specific remedies to directly affect the cortisol function.

A note about how herbal medicine is chosen: I have listed the herbs alphabetically. They are separated into the nootropic (previously called nervine) group and the adaptogen group. A nootropic is an herb that is thought to support and nourish the nerves. We do not have this concept in Western medicine. It is found commonly in herbal medicine and the nootropics are widely used for the management of anxiety. I have also attempted to describe some nuances of their activities that would guide the practitioner to choose one herb over the other.

An adaptogen is an herb that is considered to be non-toxic and a general support to the body in the management of stress. They are mostly amphoteric herbs, meaning that they can do both, stimulate *and* sedate. This characteristic makes them quite useful in the management of anxiety and of disorders related to the HPA axis. Adaptogens and nootropics are often recommended together.

Anxiety Reducing Herbs: Nootropics or Nerve Tonics

Important Note: Please remember anxiety, like depression, requires a full evaluation from a professional. Do not use any of these herbal remedies in place of professional guidance and treatment.

Bacopa (*Bacopa monnieri*). Bacopa has also been called water hyssop or Brahmi in Ayurvedic medicine. It is a bitter herb to taste, so I recommend using it as a capsule. It is useful for improvement of cognition. In my personal clinical experience, it is more useful for improving cognition and focus than anxiety even though traditionally it is recommended to reduce anxiety. It is useful in the severely mentally ill, as well as anyone who wants to improve cognition. The dose is 350 mg once or twice a day. Dr. Low Dog recommends using bacopa with gotu kola together for anxiety in children.

Blue vervain (*Verbena hastata, Verbena officianalis*). Authors Thomas Easley and Steven Horne, in their book *The Modern Herbal Dispensatory*, describe blue vervain this way: "[U]sed internally to relax the nerves and combat anxiety. It is very helpful for the nervous exhaustion from long-term stress or fanatical, hard-driving personalities and for people who suffer from neck and shoulder pain who feel like they're tied up in knots. It's helpful for women who get angry and tense before their period, and for anger in general." Drink 1–3 cups of blue vervain tea per day for anxiety reduction. I highly recommend blending this with other tasty herbs as it is quite bitter when taken alone. It is also available as an alcohol-free extract or as an alcohol-based tincture. Take 1 dropperful up to four times per day. My go-to for alcohol-free extracts is Hawaii Pharm. Do not take excessive amounts of blue vervain as it may cause nausea and vomiting.

California poppy (*Eschscholzia californica*). Unlike its relative, the opium poppy, this plant contains no opium. It is used for relaxation, sedation, and pain relief. It is consumed as a tea, which is mild, or available as a tincture, which has stronger effects. The tinctures contain alcohol so be mindful of alcohol intake. Take 1 dropperful three times a day and 2 at bedtime if needed for sleep. It is also available in alcohol-free extract form. Secrets of the Tribe sells an alcohol-free extract of California poppy combined with valerian root. California poppy is safe for children, especially those who are wound up from anxiety and not sleeping well. It will give you a positive urine test for opiates—something to keep in mind if you get drug-tested at work.

Catnip (*Nepeta cataria*). Not just for cats, catnip is a mild relaxant and calmative. This plant is helpful for young children—even infants. Serve as a tea. Never boil the herb but rather steep it. It is very effective for calming fussy babies and children when combined with fennel. Take 1 cup of tea two to three times a day. Easley and Horne describe catnip as useful for irritable bowel syndrome due to stress. It is an excellent anti-spasmodic for the colon when made with fresh leaf tincture. Easley and Horne prefer a fresh leaf glycerite of 90 percent glycerin (the standard is 70 percent). Take 1–2 teaspoons up to three times daily. Available online as a tea, as the herb, and as a glycerite.

Chamomile (*Anthemis mobilis*) and (*Matricaria recutita*). Chamomile is a mild calmative and especially helpful for all digestive problems. It is safe to use in infants and can be given in the bottle for teething and colic. It is particularly effective when used with fennel and/or caraway and lemon balm for the treatment of colic; you can also add catnip (see above). Combine all ingredients and steep for a tea. Mix ½ teaspoon of each in a cup of hot water and steep for 10 minutes. Give in small doses of 1–3 tablespoons several times a day depending on the age and need of the baby. Chamomile tea can also be made as a cold infusion. Place the chamomile in a room temperature cup of water and let it steep for 15–20 minutes. It can also be put in an ice tray and frozen. You can then put the ice cubes of chamomile in a towel and give to a baby who is teething. It is widely available over the counter and online. Do not use if there is an allergy to ragweed.

Chinese polygala (*Polygala tenuifolia, Yuan zhi*). This is a traditional Chinese medicine herb indicated for anxiety and fear. It is thought to be stronger than many other anxiolytic herbs, and it seems to be helpful for improving cognition. Large doses can cause nausea and vomiting. Do not use with gastritis, ulcers, or pregnancy. David Winston includes it in his anxiety formula (see sidebar on p. 124). It is available as granules and tinctures. Be sure not to confuse it with Senega snakeroot (*Polygala senega*), which is used for lung conditions and inflammation of the throat, nose, and chest. Follow the directions on the bottle of the product that you purchase.

Here are some formulas that you might like to try.

David Winston's Anxiety Formula

2 parts bacopa

2 parts motherwort

2 parts fresh milky oats seed

1 part blue vervain

1 part Chinese polygala

If the person's mind is racing and they cannot shut it off at night, add 2 parts Passionflower. If they have muscle tension or fly off the handle with anger add 1-part skullcap. This is best made as a combination of glycerites (alcohol-free tinctures/extracts). Purchase the glycerites individually and then combine them together. A part is simply the amount you wish to make. For example, if you want a teaspoon as your part, then you would use 2 teaspoons of bacopa, motherwort and milky oats, 1 teaspoon of blue vervain and 1 teaspoon of Chinese polygala.

From Thomas Easley *The Modern Herbal Dispensatory*, p. 152

Dr. Sharol Marie Tilgner Serenity Inducing Tea

Orange peel	*Citrus aurantium*	25–40%
Chamomile	*Matricaria recutita*	25–35%
Lavender	*Lavandula officinalis*	15–25%
Oat	*Avena sativa*	15–25%

Mix all the ingredients together except the oats. Steep the oats for 20 minutes, then add the remainder of the ingredients and let steep for 10–20 seconds. It is an aromatic tea.

Dose for acute anxiety: take 2 heaping teaspoons per cup, 4 times a day

Dose for restorative: 1 heaping teaspoon per cup, 2–3 times a day

Contraindicated in pregnancy.

From Dr. Sharol Marie Tilgner, *Herbal Medicine from the Heart of the Earth*, p. 319

Dr. Sharol Marie Tilgner Valerian Compound

Valerian	*Valeriana officinalis*	20–35%
Skullcap	*Scutellaria lateriflora*	20–35%
Kava kava	*Piper methysticum*	15–25%
Passionflower	*Passiflora incarnata*	15–25%
Oat	*Avena sativa*	10–15%

From Dr. Sharol Marie Tilgner, *Herbal Medicine from the Heart of the Earth*, p. 320

Hops (*Humulus lupulus*). Yes, I mean hops like what you find in beer. Hops is well known in herbal medicine for its calmative properties. I prefer to use glycerites (non-alcohol extracts), but the alcohol tinctures may be more potent. The dried herb, rather than the fresh, is needed for sedation. It is often mixed with other herbs, such as valerian and lemon balm, to help with sleep. It can also be used for daytime anxiety reduction. Easley and Horne describe it as "best on hot, damp people who are often overweight and red-faced with fiery personalities and have poor digestion and insomnia" (*The Modern Herbal Dispensatory*, p. 247). Take a dropper up to three times per day for anxiety and take 2 droppers at bedtime to improve sleep. My go-to for alcohol-free extracts is Hawaii Pharm.

Jatamansi (*Nardostachys jatamansi*). An herb that grows high in the Himalayan mountains, jatamansi is used in Ayurvedic medicine for the main complaint of stress and mood disorders. It is available as a pill, as a tincture or extract, and as a powder. Follow the directions on the product you purchase.

Kava kava (*Piper methysticum*). Fresh rhizomes and roots are traditionally chewed and used as a beverage in the Pacific Islands from which they come. Kava kava was initially brought to North America as a urinary anti-spasmodic. It is used currently as a mild calmative as the commercially prepared tea. Drink 2–3 cups daily for relaxation. Avoid large doses as intoxication can occur. It is initially stimulating then depressing to the nervous system. It may cause altered liver enzymes in some people, so if prolonged use is expected, check liver enzymes periodically. Avoid in pregnancy and lactation. The tea is available over the counter by the company Yogi. It is available as a supplement (pill) and also as an extract.

Lavender (*Lavandula augustifolia*). Lavender is a plant widely used for calming and relaxation. One can see fields and fields of wild lavender growing in France. It is so abundant in France that lavender is used in everything; they even have lavender ice cream. It is used in aromatherapy and fragrances as it has a pleasing scent. Lavender is also a popular essential oil. There is good evidence to support the use of lavender essential oil on the pillow to improve sleep. It is also available as a nasal inhaler and is very effective as the essential oil that goes straight into the brain. Purchase online. It is also used to relieve tension-induced headache and relax the muscles. The essential oil is often added to a bath. Do not take the essential oil internally as it is toxic quickly. However, the tea is lovely. Drink one cup, two to three times a day. It is often available commercially as a tea combined with chamomile. Traditional Medicinals makes a nice tea with this combination.

Lemon balm (*Melissa officianalis*). This herb is well known for its pleasant lemon flavor, fragrance, and uplifting effect. A member of the mint family, it is easily grown in the garden. It makes a delicious tea when freshly harvested from the garden, and produces a pleasant uplifting feeling. It has been called the "gladdening herb" as it makes one feel glad when drinking it. It is lovely as a fresh tea. Drink as desired. Lemon balm is frequently combined with other herbs. Lemon balm is also safe for children.

Linden flowers (*Tilia europea*). Sold in Europe as a beverage, it is consumed much like Americans drink a tea or coffee. It is used for its relaxing quality and its mild, sedative effects. It is helpful for reducing the effects of stress and tension. Linden flower tea has a pleasant flavor and is safe for children. Drink a cup of tea one to three times a day. Linden flowers can also be used in a bath for relaxation. Place an ounce (approximately ⅔ of a cup) of herb in a cheesecloth and put in a bath or make a strong tea (by steeping for 10–15 minutes) and add to the bath. The first time I added the linden flowers to a bath, I also added 2–3 drops of essential oil of lavender, 2–3 drops of essential oil of Roman chamomile, 2–3 drops of essential oil of black pepper, and a sprinkle of Epsom salts. While in the tub, I thought nothing was happening, but when I got out of the tub, I had some trouble with coordination, like I had had a stiff drink. I then slept for twelve hours. The effect is subtle but powerful. I recommend trying the bath on a night before a day when you have no responsibilities. Traditional Medicinals makes a tea called Nighty Night that includes many of the herbs listed here including linden flowers.

Magnolia (*Magnolia oficinalis*) and Phellodendron (*Phellodendron amurense*). The bark of both of these plants has been used in Chinese medicine for centuries. Sold commercially as Relora, a blend of extracts of *Magnolia officinalis* bark and *Phellodendron amurense* bark standardized to honokiol and berberine, respectively.[23] It was one of the first combinations of herbs that I used for the treatment of anxiety. I find it to be a safe and effective treatment. Relora can be helpful for those who overeat in response to anxiety. Follow the directions on the bottle of the product that you buy.

Motherwort (*Leonorus cardiaca*). The particular characteristic of this plant is that the leaves change in size from large at the bottom of the stem to small at the top of the stem and it is punctuated with thorns. The changes in the leaves are said to represent the changes in a woman's life and the thorns they need for clear boundaries. Motherwort is useful for women who take care of their family first and forget themselves. It is also useful for women who are in need of mothering. The name cardiaca gives you an idea that the plant may affect the heart. In fact, it is known to relieve the tachycardia (rapid heartbeat) of anxiety and of hyperthyroidism. Motherwort is a bitter herb, so it is also useful for improving digestion. Most prefer to take it as a capsule or a glycerite because of its bitterness. As a tea, take 2–3 ounces, two to three times a day. Follow the directions on the bottle of the product that you buy. It should not be used during pregnancy.

Passionflower (*Passiflora incarnata*). Passionflower is a widely used, common herb found in commercial preparations of tea. In spite of its name, it's the leaves of the plant that are used. Passionflower is commonly mixed with other herbs; you will often see it mixed with lemon balm and lavender, among others. It has a common indication of improving sleep disturbed by worry or nightmares. It is helpful for those who cannot turn off their thinking. It may calm the palpitations caused by anxiety. It also may be helpful for bruxism (teeth grinding) when mixed with skullcap. It is very safe for the old and the young. Consume as a tea for a relaxing night's sleep. You may drink up to 3 cups daily.

Poria (*Wolfiporia extensa, Poria spirit*). Poria is a lesser-known medicinal mushroom, but it is extremely popular in China and is found in 10 percent of all Chinese formulas. Poria is found under many names in commercial products, but the one I recommend for anxiety and insomnia is *Poria cocos* known as Fu shen. In Chinese medicine, the shen is the spirit and when unquiet, *Poria* will calm it. Interestingly, it also is used as a treatment for the digestive system. *Poria* is a unique mushroom in that it does not form the typical stem and cap that most mushrooms form, but rather its mycelia are formed into a ball underground that resembles a coconut; hence the name *Poria cocos*. An alcohol-free version is made by Hawaii Pharm. Take 1 dropperful at night before bed and if there is any hangover feeling the next day, reduce the dose. It is very calming and works fairly quickly. Do not take before using heavy machinery or driving.

Skullcap (*Scutellaria lateriflora*). Known for relaxing qualities, skullcap is an excellent nootropic, tonic herb that relaxes nervousness. Take during the day as a tea or tincture and you may not need additional herbs to help you sleep. The glycerite of this herb is also helpful for anxious, yappy dogs. They love it and will lick it right off the dropper. You can find this as a tea, a tincture, or an alcohol-free extract. Follow directions on the bottle. Skullcap is often mixed with other herbs for relaxation and can be found in many commercial preparations. A common companion herb is passionflower. You can put a spoonful, or a teabag of each tea in a cup of hot water, steep, strain, and drink.

St. John's wort (*Hypericum perforatum*). St. John's wort is a well-known and widely used herb and may be familiar to the reader. It has the reputation of being an anti-depressant. It is less well known for its pain-relieving properties (especially used topically) and its relaxing qualities. St. John's wort comes as a tea and has been consumed as a tea for centuries as a folk medicine. It has been used to relax and calm the system and to improve sleep. It has been shown to relieve depressed mood in a mild to moderate depression. It is very effective as a topical treatment for any nerve pain and for muscle sprain and strain.

The limiting factor in using St. John's wort is its drug interaction. St. John's wort stimulates the enzyme that breaks down many medications, making those medications ineffective. Hormones and anti-rejection drugs used in transplants are common drug interactions and the herb should be avoided. Check with a medical professional before consuming if you are taking any prescription medication. You can find St. John's wort as an herb to make into a tea, as a commercially prepared tea, or as a capsule.

Valerian (*Valeriana officianalis*). Valerian is a popular herb that may be known to the reader as a sleep remedy but was used historically for nervous stomach. Valerian is used as an anti-anxiety herb and is especially helpful for those whose anxiety affects their digestive tract. The dried herb has the smell of dirty gym socks and is quite unpleasant. Christopher Hobbs describes the smell of the fresh root and the essential oil as a "sweet, musky odor that is quite pleasant."[24] However, he may be alone in that assessment. If taken as a supplement pill, take 500 mg three times per day to relieve anxiety.

Valerian is often sold in combination with other nootropic herbs in the marketplace. Secrets of the Tribe sells an alcohol-free extract of the combination of California poppy and valerian root. The smell is quite strong. Valerian can also be found in combination with hops as a supplement and also as a bath oil. Because of its strong aromatics, I recommend taking this herb as a supplement over any other method unless you do not mind the scent (some people do not mind it and may actually like it). Valerian is widely available over the counter. Follow the directions on the bottle of the product that you purchase. Be aware that there are a few people for whom valerian has an opposite effect and they will be stimulated by it.

Wild lettuce (*Lactuca virosa*). A lesser-known plant used for its relaxant and analgesic properties. Wild lettuce is used to relieve pain and to impart relaxation to both the mind and the body. It is helpful for improving sleep disturbed by anxiety and worry or pain in the body. The herbal tea is bitter and is best combined with other herbs. It is commercially available as a glycerite (alcohol-free extract) from Hawaii Pharm. Take a dropperful two to four times a day to relieve anxiety.

Wild oats (*Avena fatua, A. sativa*). This plant is used as a nerve support that is specific for exhaustion due to depression. It may also be helpful for withdrawal from addictions. The tincture needs to be made from a fresh herb that has a milky exudate. You can make a tea and drink several times per day for relaxation and improvement in sleep routine. Wild oats are very helpful for wound up children that are hyperactive due to anxiety. Make the tea and the child can drink it freely. An alcohol-free extract can also be mixed in a juice. Most products are sold in the United States as *Avena sativa* and most often in the form of milky seeds. The milky seeds are used in the same way as described above. Herb Pharm carries an alcohol-free tincture. Not for use in pregnancy.

Wood betony (*Stachys officianalis*). A much lesser-known herb but one that is a personal favorite is wood betony. It is very helpful for reducing muscle tension due to anxiety and overwork. It is particularly helpful for the headache immediately following a head injury or trauma. Wood betony brews to a pleasant tasting tea with a vanilla aftertaste, and I recommend adding a little vanilla to the tea for flavor. Drink 1 cup two to three times daily. It is also available as a tincture or an extract. Follow the directions on the bottle of the product you purchase.

Adaptogens

I learned how to think about adaptogens (which ones to pick, how to match an adaptogen to a person) from Dr. Tieraona Low Dog. She has specific ideas about what these herbs mean to her, and those ideas frame my thinking in a clinical setting. The nuances of the various adaptogens come directly from her and I give her all the credit. The supportive research and combination recommendations come from the book, *Adaptogens, Herbs for Strength, Stamina and Stress Relief,* by David Winston, RH (AHG) and Steven Maimes (Healing Arts Press, Rochester, Vermont, 2007 and 2019). Adaptogens and nootropics are often recommended together.

Ashwagandha (*Withania somnifera*). This herb has been used in Ayurvedic medicine for supporting the HPA axis and the thyroid, increasing iron in the iron deficient, and for relaxation and improved sleep. Ashwagandha is the most sedating of the adaptogens and as such is useful in the management of anxiety. It was used for iron deficiency anemia before we had iron replacement capacity, and also to support the thyroid before we had thyroid supplementation. It has also been shown to be useful in the treatment of some cancers and is used in cancer protocols in India. It has been shown to reduce tumor size and improve immune function. It is also used to enhance both male and female sexuality, including sperm count and motility, and is considered an aphrodisiac. It has been used to improve sleep and cognitive fogginess. Interestingly, it is also used for a wide variety of topical ailments.[25] David Winston describes using ashwagandha (*Withania somnifera*) in conjunction with white peony (*Paeonia lactiflora*) and black cohosh root (*Actae racemosa*) for the physical pain of fibromyalgia, muscles cramps in the neck and back, and for joint pain due to osteoarthritis. Given the debilitating effect of chronic pain on someone's life, these remedies may bring great relief to both body and mind. The herb is available as a tincture, as an alcohol-free extract (Nature's

Way and Hawaii Pharm), and also as the raw herb to be made into a tea. Dr. Low Dog likes this herb made with almond milk instead of water. Simmer for 15 minutes and add cardamom and some sweetener. Drink a half a cup three times per day. Personally, I find the taste to be unpleasantly bitter and prefer to consume it as a tea when mixed with other pleasant tasting herbs. It is also available as a capsule. Take 400–500 mg twice daily. It is considered safe but should not be used in hemochromatosis (iron-storing disease) or in hyperthyroidism.

Eleuthero (*Eleuthero senticosus*). Formerly known as Siberian ginseng, eleuthero normalizes the HPA axis. It is good to use for those who gorge on carbs, especially when anxious, and for those who don't sleep well and regularly have dark circles under their eyes. Russian studies have found that people who use eleuthero with *Andrographis paniculata*, took fewer sick days. Studies also show a decrease in bone marrow suppression from chemo and radiation cancer treatment. It is best used for those who work hard, play hard, and hardly sleep. It is available as a tincture, an alcohol-free extract, as a tea, and as a supplement. I like to make this tea with almond milk and cardamom and cinnamon. Simmer for 20–30 minutes, steep for an hour, strain, and drink up to 3 cups per day. Dr. Low Dog believes it is not necessary to drink it every day, but several times per week will help. It is also appropriate for long-term use.

Holy basil (*Ocimum tenuiflorum [synonym O. sanctum] and O. gratissimum*). In Ayurvedic medicine, holy basil, also known as Tulsi, is believed to be a rasayana, meaning an herb that nourishes and provides long life. In India it is highly revered and considered sacred. It is also used in cooking as a spice and is known to be helpful in relieving gastrointestinal upset. It also has a calming effect on the psyche with an improvement in mental clarity. It is useful in the treatment of anxiety as it is known to lower cortisol levels by blunting cortisol releasing hormone at the pituitary. It is particularly helpful for brain fog from any cause (menopause, head injury, etc.). Holy basil can be consumed as a tea, a spice, a capsule, or a tincture/extract. It is commonly found in combination with other herbs. For the tea, use 1 teaspoon of dried leaves per 8-ounce cup of hot water. Let steep 5–10 minutes and drink 1–3 cups daily. If you purchase a tincture or an extract, follow the directions on the bottle. Avoid in pregnancy and when trying to conceive.

A personal note on holy basil: I have a great deal of respect for the potency of holy basil. I once made a tea from this herb and it had such a profound effect on my psyche, with intense dreams and an almost hallucinatory experience, that I sent it back to the company to be analyzed for purity. However, it was pure, and every time I drink holy basil alone, I have the same experience. Therefore, I recommend using holy basil in conjunction with other herbs rather than alone.

Panax ginseng. Ginseng blunts the response of adrenocorticotropin hormone (ACTH) at the adrenal glands. It is best to use for those with hyperarousal, difficulty staying asleep, and early morning awakening. There is controversy over what the ginsenosides (the constituents thought to be the most active) do and where they are found in the plant. According to Dr. Low Dog the root is the most balanced in function, so use only roots from reputable manufacturers that can tell you where the plant comes from, harvest to sale. Ginseng is used for those who have adrenal depletion (dark circles under the eyes, and allergies), insomnia, emotional distress, depression, and poor memory. It is also thought to improve nitric oxide (NO), so there is some research that shows it improves erectile dysfunction. It is a good idea to take only in the morning. Choose Asian ginseng for those with cold hands and feet who are sick a lot, and American ginseng for those in the resistance phase of the stress cycle or who have melancholic depression. Both types of ginseng are available as the raw root to be made into a tea, tincture, and capsule. Make the tea as a decoction: Simmer 1–2 teaspoons of ground herb for ½ an hour and then steep it for an additional hour. Drink 1–2 cups daily. Take 400–500 mg of herb, 2 capsules, twice a day. If you are a type A personality and very driven, large quantities of Asian ginseng will make you more anxious. It is a good idea to avoid coffee while taking Asian ginseng. There is a drug interaction with coumadin, and it should be avoided. Also, ginseng may increase the strength of MAOI anti-depressants, so be sure to be monitored by your physician if you take this medication.

Rhodiola (*Rhodiola rosea*). Rhodiola, also known as Arctic root, has a long history of being used to support energy, increase endurance, and reduce fatigue. It is very well studied and has been used for decades in Russia, Scandinavia, Tibet, and Germany. As the name implies, it grows in cold climates. It has been used to improve focus and performance. There is an open UCLA study that shows rhodiola was helpful for reducing symptoms of generalized anxiety disorder after administration for ten weeks. The sample size was small but after I heard about this study, I had two patients in a row tell me how rhodiola lessened their anxiety. Most of the research has been on the use of rhodiola for attention deficit disorder and depression, as well as fatigue. Personally, I find the herb stimulating and drying. In excess it will cause dry mouth and constipation. It is contraindicated in bipolar disorder due to its stimulating property. Since it is also drying, use caution if you have dry eyes, dry mouth (Sjögren's syndrome), or very dry skin. It is available as a tincture, extract, tea, or capsule. The capsules should be standardized to 3–5 percent rosavins and 1 percent salidrosides. Take 2–4 capsules daily. Follow the directions on the bottle if you buy a tincture or extract. If drinking the tea, make a decoction by simmering the cut and sifted roots for 15 minutes, then let steep 45 minutes. Drink 1–2 cups daily.

In chapter 5, "The Cortisol Connection," there is a table of commercially sold products readily available. You may be interested in revisiting that table.

Herbs Helpful to Children

Hsiao yao wan (Free and Easy Wanderer). This is a well-known Chinese patented herbal remedy for children who are angry, acting out, and irritable. Give 5–8 tablets daily for several weeks. This product is a combination of 8 herbs: Bupleurum, Dong qui, White peony root, White atracylodes, Pora (Fu ling), Peppermint, Quick-fried ginger root (Pao jian) and Licorice root. Avoid in pregnancy.

Red clover blossom. This herb has the added benefit of detoxification as well as a calmative. Use 1 teaspoon of herb per cup of water to make a tea. Take half a cup twice a day.

You will notice that all of these herbs recommend multiple doses throughout the day. In my clinical experience, that is impractical. Most people can manage one or two doses throughout the day, but the mid-day dose is usually forgotten.

The evening dose is also sometimes forgotten. The frequent dosing of the herbal remedies implies that they are short acting. Taking the time out of a busy day to brew a cup of tea or make a decoction is even more demanding. I often recommend the act of brewing a cup of tea *and sitting down and drinking it* as a meditation and break from the busyness of the day. The supplement (pill) form of all these remedies may be more useful because they can be taken in combination and the patient can double up on the dose at night to make it easier to get the recommended dosage.

Essential Oils for Anxiety

Major essential oil companies sell blends that are meant to reduce anxiety. There are also many individual essential oils that are known to have good efficacy against anxiety disorders. Essential oils are used for their aroma; as an anxiety treatment the oil is often inhaled through a nasal inhaler or used in an essential oil diffuser. Some essential oils can be used on the skin, either directly or with a carrier oil. Some can be placed on a cotton ball and put in the pillowcase to help reduce anxiety that interferes with sleep.

The most widely known oil to reduce anxiety is lavender. Inhaling the lavender oil is the most direct way to get the oil into the brain, and has been found to have an immediate effect. Lavender can be inhaled as needed.

My friend and colleague, Inga Wieser, N.D., M.S., M.A. APAIA, MH, is the current president of the Alliance of International Aromatherapists, an expert in essential oils, and a master herbalist. She uses the following essential oils for anxiety reduction: lavender, bergamot, geranium, ylang, frankincense, rose, cedarwood, sweet marjoram, and jasmine. For panic attacks, jasmine and patchouli can be helpful. The way she uses these essential oils is as oil blends, which are made specifically for the individual. If you are interested in the use of essential oils, I recommend making an appointment with a professional to make a remedy just for you.

Other Treatments for Anxiety

I want to briefly mention some other treatments I use and recommend to my patients.

Resistance Training

There are numerous articles that describe the benefits of resistance training for anxiety. It appears that lower weight resistance training is more beneficial than heavy weight or intense workouts. Resistance training builds strength and muscle size. It requires some equipment—weights or resistance bands are the most common pieces of equipment utilized. The way to determine the amount of weight needed is to lift the heaviest weight you can possibly lift just once. Then take 15 percent to 17 percent of that amount and use that much weight as your workout. For example, if you can lift a 30-pound dumbbell one time, then a 5-pound weight would be your ideal. There does seem to be a threshold of resistance that is necessary for effective anxiety relief. Even one resistance workout can lower acute anxiety. This is helpful to know for the management of acute anxiety episodes that may occur and overlie a chronic anxiety disorder.

Cognitive Behavioral Therapy (CBT)

Therapy is often the cornerstone of treatment. Reframing the thoughts and beliefs that trigger the anxiety in the first place is crucial to long-term success. I discussed this type of therapy under the treatment for depression. See chapter 11.

The Alpha Stim

An FDA approved medical device which is indicated for the treatment of anxiety, depression, insomnia, and chronic pain. This device clips to the earlobes and stimulates the alpha waves of the brain which are relaxing. It is a most convenient treatment modality. Find more information from www.alpha-stim.com.

Neurofeedback

This is a technique that utilizes a computerized electroencephalogram (EEG) to map the brain waves of the brain. Then the visual system is stimulated so the brain waves can either be stimulated or quieted depending on the need of the patient. This treatment requires going to a practitioner's office twice weekly for treatment. There are some neurofeedback systems that are available for home use. My experience is with the Loretta in-office system. To find a neurofeedback provider in your area, go to: www.bcia.org.

An Herbalist's Approach to Treating Anxiety

Kelly is a thirty-two-year-old woman who had her first suicidal thought of walking out of a window at the age of thirteen and depression has been part of her life ever since. She developed anxiety in high school when she felt anxious around other people and at sporting events in which she was a participant. When her anxiety heightens, she feels her heart race, she feels the need to escape and leave a room because she perceives it is closing in on her, and she may have a full-blown panic attack. Most bothersome to her, however, are memory and focus problems which interfere with her ability to maintain a job. She also complains of difficulty with sleep, and in the past year had been formally diagnosed with sleep apnea and prescribed a CPAP machine. She does not wear her sleep apnea mask because it is uncomfortable.

In taking a full history, I determined that there was a hormonal component to Kelly's depression. Her depression began at the onset of puberty, and she told me she suffered irregular, heavy, and painful periods. These periods were most likely anovulatory (without ovulation). Had she been my patient back then, my approach would have been to regulate her periods with the herb *Vitex agnus-castus*. However, her pediatrician placed her on oral contraceptives and her periods normalized. By the time she came to me, she was no longer taking oral contraceptives and her menstruation was normal in both regularity and flow. But she still had fluctuations in mood during her cycle, and I suspected there was an ongoing hormonal piece at play.

Herbs for Treating Anxiety

The herbs I recommended for Kelly are listed here:

For depression and anxiety: St. John's wort (*Hypericum perforatum*). This herb is excellent for depressed mood, anxiety reduction and for sleep. At the time she presented to me she was not taking any medication, so St. John's wort was safe for her to take. I recommended 900 mg at bedtime.

I also strongly recommended that she use the CPAP machine and to revisit the sleep doctor to get a more comfortable mask. It is very hard to improve depressed mood when there is sleep apnea in the background.

We also discussed the use of lamotrigine, a seizure medication used in psychiatry as a mood stabilizer, to stabilize the moods and improve the depression. She chose to add this to her regimen. It is safe for her to take with the St. John's wort.

For hormonal support: *Vitex agnus-castus*. This will increase the progesterone in the last half of her menstrual cycle and should alleviate anxiety. I recommended one 400 mg capsule (from Nature's Way with the green top) daily.

Black cohosh (*Actea racemosa*). This is to improve the depression and level the mood. The dose is one 540 mg capsule, twice daily, from Nature's Way (bottle with the green top).

Adaptogen: *Panax ginseng*, Red Korean. The red color is from steaming the root, but white is the natural color at harvesting. Panax ginseng is perfect for her due to her insomnia, emotional distress, depression, and poor memory. This is a stimulating herb and should help with her difficulty with focus.

The rest of the recommendations included cognitive behavioral therapy, the alpha stim, neurofeedback, hyperbaric oxygen therapy (since she had also had a concussion), the interactive metronome (to help with focus), omega 3 fatty acids, and a multivitamin. She already had a healthy diet and a good exercise program, which I encouraged her to continue. She also had a regular meditation program she performed daily. I recommended that she stop smoking marijuana on a regular basis as it decreases blood flow to the prefrontal cortex and decreases motivation and focus. I also recommended her alcohol consumption follow the recommendations made by the Academy of Addiction Psychiatry for a total of seven drinks in a week and no more than two per day.

We also discussed the possibility of more aggressive depression treatments such as transcranial magnetic stimulation (TMS) and IV ketamine therapy if needed, but fortunately her compliance with all of the above resulted in significant improvement.

PART IV

HERBAL MEDICINE FOR ADD/ADHD

• •

13

DEFICITS IN ATTENTION AND FOCUS

Attention deficit disorder (ADD) and attention deficit hyperactivity disorder (ADHD) are real psychiatric problems with profound consequences for the person who has them and for their families. ADD/ADHD are a syndrome—a constellation of symptoms that appear together, and as such, the causes and presentations are varied.

ADD, inattentive type, is characterized by inattention, easy distractibility, lack of focus, difficulty with organization and time management, and trouble completing tasks. ADHD includes all the symptoms of the inattentive type *plus* impulsivity and the inability to sit still, be quiet, think before speaking or acting, or wait one's turn.

Attention deficit disorder is classified as a neurodevelopmental disorder. By definition the disorder is one of the young because that is when the brain is developing, and the disorder occurs. Research has shown that in children with attention deficit disorder, the motor cortex of the brain develops faster (accounting for the hyperactivity) and the prefrontal cortex portion of the brain (the part for focus and attention) lags behind.[26] Research has also found evidence of oxidative stress

147

and oxidation of purines, the building blocks of DNA, in the brains of children with ADD. Oxidative stress and oxidation of purines are processes that develop reactive oxygen species (ROS) with associated damage to the DNA. [27, 28] You may know ROS by the term "free radicals" for which antioxidant supplements are recommended. These free radicals are causing damage to the growing brain at the level of the gene, the DNA itself.

Although ADD, as a disorder, typically presents initially in childhood, those children grow up and bring their ADD along with them into adulthood, and many people are diagnosed with ADD for the first time as an adult. Attention and focus are closely related to memory and cognition. Those with the disorder may have difficulty with memory and poor thinking, including poor performance in school and at work. Some people who are exceptionally intelligent are able to compensate for their brain difficulties and be successful and do well in school and work without treatment.

In this chapter, I want to share my experience in treating ADD by using non-pharmacological means. Most of my experience has been with the inattentive type. I have also treated the other subtypes described below. I will also discuss some of the different ways the disorder can present and address some of the controversies surrounding the diagnosis and treatments.

Inattention and Lack of Focus

In my experience, there is nothing more effective than stimulant medication for improving attention and focus, unless the inattention is due to or mixed with anxiety. If the inattention is due to anxiety or overactivity of the brain, a stimulant may worsen the symptoms. The treatment in the case of anxiety-driven inattention is to treat the anxiety. (See chapter 12 for anxiety treatment options.) Sometimes the anxiety and classic inattention occur together and both the attention and the anxiety need to be treated. One benefit of the SPECT scans we utilize at the Amen Clinics is their ability to clearly delineate the cause of the inattention. If the SPECT scan clearly shows a decrease in blood flow to the prefrontal cortex and basal ganglia, that indicates the inattention will respond to stimulation that increases dopamine (stimulant medication or stimulating herbs). The SPECT scan can also identify the overactivity of the brain indicative of anxiety. This makes it much easier for the clinician to choose the appropriate treatment.

There are times when patients do not want stimulant medications, or for some reason it is not appropriate for them to have the stimulant medication (for example, prior stimulant abuse), so there is a need for natural remedies to improve focus. I try to set appropriate expectations; the truth is that herbal remedies do *not* work as well as the stimulant medication in increasing focus. But they can be helpful. Also, the number of pills that one has to take when taking herbal medicine for ADD may be greater than the number of pills required from a stimulant.

Diagnostic Approaches to ADD/ADHD

Because ADD/ADHD is a constellation of symptoms making up a syndrome, it can be more difficult to diagnose. There are some practitioners who have recognized subsets of ADD/ADHD. I would like to review the work of two practitioners who have addressed this issue: Dr. Scott Shannon and Dr. Daniel Amen, both of whom take the approach to ADD/ADHD much further than just prescribing a stimulant medication. For a comprehensive discussion of the types and associated treatments please go to the books, *Mental Health for the Whole Child* by Dr. Shannon and *Healing ADD* by Dr. Daniel Amen.

Dr. Scott Shannon

Dr. Shannon is not convinced that ADD is an illness, but rather a result of underlying metabolic derangements. He wants to know, "What is going on with the whole child?" In his book, *Mental Health for the Whole Child,* he discusses seven different subtypes of ADD. You will see that some of the subtypes are based on metabolic problems and some on environmental disturbances.

Type 1: Anxious and over-focused. The inattention is driven by anxiety, but people with this type of ADD are still able to focus on one thing that is of interest. The treatment approach is to treat the underlying anxiety.

Type 2: Food allergies and gut imbalance. As I discussed in chapter 4, "The Gut-Brain Connection," the gut plays a significant role in all mental health. Dr. Shannon understands this and recommends checking for gastrointestinal inflammation when ADD/ADHD presents itself. Given the research listed above regarding the oxidative injury found associated with ADD/ADHD, it would make sense that poor diet, food allergies, or other reasons for gastrointestinal inflammation would be present. Treating the underlying dietary indiscretions would be the appropriate treatment.

Type 3: Mitochondrial issues and developmental delays. The mitochondria are the energy centers of the cell. If they are ill, the characteristic symptom will be a lack of activity and energy. These patients may have decreased attention, but usually have accompanying fatigue, especially in the later part of the day. The treatment for this condition would be to support the mitochondria with whole foods, carnitine, CoQ10 and medicinal mushrooms such as reishi (*Ganoderma lucidum*), lion's mane (*Leonotis Leonurus*), and/or turkey tail (*Trametes versicolor*). Consider sleep apnea in this type.

Type 4: Classic ADHD. This type comprises what one typically thinks of when thinking about ADD: hyperactive, can't sit still, trouble with focus and completing tasks, tends to be a daredevil, seeks conflict. Dr. Shannon's approach for this type is mostly environmental. Allow the child to be active in school, give them lots of structure, and limit video games that are very stimulating to the brain.

Type 5: Angry and oppositional. These are generally unhappy children. They are characterized by conflict, mood lability, and erratic behavior. They tend to be worse at home. Look for family abuse and mental illness. Dr. Shannon recommends avoiding stimulants with this type.

Type 6: Environmental issues. This type is characterized by chaos in the home. Often the parent (or parents) is overwhelmed and the kid turns to video games, often violent ones. Often there is sleep disruption. Dr. Shannon recommends structure and avoiding stimulant medication.

Type 7: Apathy and learning issues. Often this type of presentation is one of avoidance—avoiding school, avoiding reading, avoiding academics in general. Dr. Shannon's approach to this type is to avoid stimulant medication in high doses and to recognize that it loses value over time. This child may require a small school with a lot of structure but one that allows for his/ her abilities to be supported.

Dr. Daniel Amen

Dr. Daniel Amen also identifies seven types of ADD, but they are based on SPECT brain scans. I find the brain scans to be very helpful in being able to identify the subtype of ADD and to pick the appropriate treatment. The approach will always include diet, exercise, optimizing labs (such as iron, copper, and others), as well as family and academic structure. Two SPECT scans are performed, one at rest and the other, a concentration scan, is performed after a computerized test called The Conner's test, which demands attention to complete.

Type 1: Classic ADD. This is the most familiar type of ADD: difficulty with focus, attention, and hyperactivity. This type is also the type most studied, with imaging studies outside of the Amen Clinic. The SPECT findings are low blood flow to the underside of the prefrontal cortex, the cerebellum, and the basal ganglia during concentration. This type is often responsive to stimulant medications. The best diet to go along with this ADD type is high protein, low carbohydrate. Regular aerobic exercise is an essential component of the treatment plan.

Type 2: Inattentive ADD. The SPECT findings are the same as the classic ADD but the patient is not hyperactive. This type is often responsive to stimulant medications. The improvement in function can be dramatic. In addition to the stimulant medication, a high protein/low carbohydrate diet and regular aerobic exercise is recommended. This type and type 1 both respond well to alternative treatments. L-tyrosine, an amino acid precursor to dopamine, and DL-phenylalanine can be helpful (see below). Also the herbal treatments listed below can be valuable as well.

Type 3: Over-focused ADD. The SPECT scan of this type shows the telltale signs of low blood flow to the underside of the brain including the prefrontal cortex, the cerebellum, and the basal ganglia. However, what is also present is overactivity of the anterior cingulate gyrus. The anterior cingulate gyrus is what we call the brain's gear-shifter. This overactivity is associated with symptoms of trouble shifting attention (getting stuck), cognitive inflexibility, and excessive negative thoughts. This type of ADD often does poorly with stimulant medication and requires that the brain is quieted first before stimulant medication is administered, although stimulant medication may or may not be utilized. Dr. Amen has found this pattern is often present in the children and grandchildren of alcoholics. The diet for this type is quality protein, complex carbohydrate (an apple versus a sticky bun), and aerobic exercise. Aerobic exercise boosts serotonin and dopamine. Serotonin calms the brain and dopamine is stimulating to the prefrontal cortex, improving focus.

Type 4: Temporal lobe ADD. On the SPECT scans of this type there are the usual telltale signs of ADD: the decrease in blood flow to the underside of the brain in the prefrontal cortex, the cerebellum, and the basal ganglia, but there is also a decrease in the blood flow of the temporal lobes. The symptoms present in this type are the ADD symptoms of inattention, distractibility, and disorganization, but also dark thoughts, mood lability, memory difficulties and learning disabilities, short and long-term memory, visual and auditory processing, and the processing of language. There may or may not be hyperactivity. An effective treatment for the temporal lobe irritability is an antiepileptic medication (lamotrigine, oxcarbazepine, carbamazepine) used in psychiatry to stabilize moods and calm the brain. Sometimes, after the seizure medication has calmed the brain, there may be residual inattention. In that case, a stimulant medication is warranted and effective. Natural treatment alternatives to the seizure medication are GABA and other supplements that are calming such as L-theanine and magnesium. The herbal stimulants listed below are appropriate here as well.

Type 5 Limbic ADD. Again, we have the telltale signs of ADD on the SPECT scan, the low blood flow to the undersurface of the brain, the prefrontal cortex, the basal ganglia, and the cerebellum; however, we also have an increase in activity of the limbic system, the thalamus, and hypothalamus that is seen in both the active scans (baseline and concentration). In this type there are symptoms of hopelessness, worthlessness, social isolation, and fatigue. There may be depression as well. The significant identifying feature here is the tendency to low energy, negative self-talk, and the feeling of being overwhelmed by stress in life in addition to the tendency toward easy distractibility and difficulty with focus.

Anti-depressants and stimulants alone often make the patient feel more moody and depressed. It is important to encourage relaxation first before stimulating the brain. Essential oils, supplements, and herbal medicine for relaxation can be helpful. *Bacopa monnieri* and *Gotu kola* both encourage relaxation and also improve focus. Lemon balm is uplifting and improves focus, as does holy basil. Working with changing the mindset, keeping options open, and avoiding all or nothing thinking are helpful. Following a diet of healthy proteins and fats and fewer carbohydrates is helpful for underlying support of the mood. Animals with wings, such as turkey or chicken, are naturally high in the amino acid tryptophan. Tryptophan is a precursor to serotonin and encourages the brain in the direction of serotonin production. Consuming turkey and chicken can increase the tryptophan level and improve the mood.

Type 6: Ring of fire ADD. The SPECT scan findings of this type are a distinctive picture. There is overactivity in the parietal lobes, the temporal lobes, the right and left prefrontal cortex, and the anterior cingulate gyrus, forming a picture of a ring of hyperactivity on the scan. The characteristic ADD symptoms of inattention and distractibility are present along with irritability, being overly sensitive to sounds and touch, oppositional behavior, and having mood cycles. This type of ADD may be due to infection or an inflammatory process. The use of stimulants and serotonergic medications can often worsen this type of brain pattern when used alone. Since this pattern is often from inflammation, an emphasis on cleaning up the gut is important; an elimination diet to rule out food allergies, removing inflammatory foods, and focusing on healthful, whole food eating is important to quiet this type of inflammation. A thorough workup for any infections in the rest of the body that may be contributing to the inflammation in the brain is important as well. The treatment is to use supplements, natural products to calm the overactivity of the brain, or to use antiepileptic medications. The antiepileptic medications such as lamotrigine or oxcarbazepine can be very helpful for a patient with this brain type. Once the brain is quieted, if a stimulant is needed it can be added with good success.

Type 7: Anxious ADD. The characteristic of this type is the overactivity of the basal ganglia accompanied by a decrease in the undersurface of the prefrontal cortex and the cerebellum. The symptoms of this type include a lack of attention, distractibility, anxiety, and tension. There is also the tendency to freeze in a crisis, predict the worst, and have social anxiety. Many ADD patients seek conflict to increase the dopamine levels in the brain. This particular type of ADD patient does not seek conflict but rather avoids anxiety-producing situations. When someone is anxious it is difficult for their thinking to land on a particular thought and follow it to conclusion. There may also be complaints of memory difficulties for the same reason.

The treatment approach for this ADD type is to reduce the anxiety, preferably with supplements and natural products. *Bacopa monnieri* and *gotu kola* are good examples of calming agents that also improve focus. Holy basil is also known to calm the brain and improve focus. Any of the herbs or natural remedies listed in the anxiety chapter would apply here. The diet that is most helpful for this brain type is low carbohydrate and high protein. There is also a place for therapy, meditation, and deep relaxation techniques.

Controversies Surrounding Diagnosis and Treatment

There are some practitioners who do not believe that ADD/ADHD is an actual disorder. This is most unfortunate for those who have it. Many think that ADD/ADHD is over-diagnosed and every high-energy child is given the diagnosis. Many think that children are being prescribed addictive, powerful medications unnecessarily. Many think that ADD/ADHD is an

American diagnosis, not found in other countries. There is a great deal of concern because the prevalence of ADD is increasing. Some think the prevalence is increasing simply due to over-diagnosis and the pressure from the schools to force medication on children. All of this controversy can leave people who need help without a diagnosis and treatment.

Why the Incidence of ADD Is Increasing

In the past decade, the number of cases of ADD/ADHD diagnosed in the United States has increased more than 30 percent, and it is estimated that 10 percent of American children have ADD.[29] This number is much higher than in other developed countries and leads some to argue that ADD/ADHD is overly diagnosed in this country.[30] Undoubtedly, there is a high demand for focus and attention in our society. Although many complaints of impaired attention and focus are caused by ADD/ADHD, some of the complaints I receive for improvement of focus I believe are more for cognitive and performance enhancement rather than true attention deficit disorder. Still, I do believe we are seeing an actual increase in cases. Below are some of the theories why this is so.

Social Policy and Pharmaceutical Influence

Stephen Hinshaw clearly demonstrates that the presence of ADD/ADHD is a worldwide phenomenon and the prevalence is 5 percent to 7 percent across countries with compulsory education.[31] He makes the interesting argument that the human brain did not evolve to attain skills sitting in a classroom. He states, "From this perspective, the confluence of biological vulnerability with psychosocial and cultural forces produces the phenomenon termed ADHD, with compulsory education serving as the triggering social factor."[32] It would be of interest to research countries where education is not so structured or compulsory to see if perhaps the development of ADD/ADHD would be less apparent or less prevalent if the individual was able to develop, grow, and learn in their respective styles.

Many are concerned about the pressure from pharmaceutical ads for medication and the pressure from schools on families to medicate their children. This pressure leads to an increase in ADD diagnoses and an increase in prescriptions for stimulant medications. Because ADD is considered a disability and medication is covered by insurance, school systems will recommend the diagnosis be made and the children medicated.

Electronics

The influence of video games, television, and the Internet cannot be overstated. All of these electronics have a particular wavelength of light and a constant flashing of that light (the way the screen refreshes itself), which is very stimulating to the brain. The rate at which the flash occurs will have a profound effect on what the observer is feeling. If the rate is slow, you will become mesmerized and sleepy. If the rate is fast you can develop anxiety and be alert. There is a great deal of research being done currently on the detrimental effects of the electromagnetic waves on the brain. I have a direct experience with the effect of these wavelengths. I was sound asleep on a plane when I felt like something was tugging at me and it awakened me from my deep sleep. The person sitting next to me had turned on his laptop. I am certain it was the electromagnetic waves being emitted from his screen that woke me.

Think about what that electromagnetic effect is doing to the brains of children who expose themselves to it for hours a day. We can't avoid screens. We need them for work, school, and more, so I encourage everyone I know to wear blue light blocking glasses and keep their computer and phone screens on as dark a setting as possible. Screen time is unavoidable in our digital world, but these precautions can help.

Television is passive, presenting all you need to know without requiring that you think or problem solve. Television tends to make people passive and intellectually lazy.

Video games are highly addictive for some kids. They will play the games incessantly to the detriment of all other activities. They will become aggressive and argue if the game is taken away. I had one family tell me that their son would break into a locked safe to get to the video game. At times, parents are forced to employ draconian measures to remove the influence of video games from the child. Many parents are not willing to do what is necessary because it is so painful. The more kids are playing video games, watching TV, spending time on their phones and social media, the less well they do in school and the worse their attention becomes.

Adults can be addicted to games as well. I was on a hotel elevator with an employee of the hotel. He was playing a game on his phone. I commented on it and he told me that his boss had threatened to fire him for playing the game on his phone because he played so much that it interfered with his work. Yet here he was, playing the game at work. He could not even ride an elevator for a matter of a few minutes without playing that game. He no doubt had an addiction.

Nutritional Effect

Tying in the gut effect, another issue for ADD is poor nutrition. ADD kids and adults tend to consume large amounts of processed foods, sugars, and sodas. Many parents with ADD kids will tell you that when their kids eat sugar, or processed foods like pizza, and drink sodas they will be "bouncing off the walls." Diets such as the elimination diet, the Feingold diet (avoiding food additives), and anti-inflammatory diets have been recommended for both autism spectrum disorder and for ADD. The consumption of highly processed foods is damaging to the gut causing inflammation in the gut wall leading to immune distress in the body as a whole and damaging to the gut microbiome.

Research on the gut microbiome is a burgeoning field with more than seven thousand published scientific articles a month on the topic. The microbiome is made up of the billions of bacterial organisms in the body. The ones in the gut are responsible for helping our food digest. They interact with hormones, make our vitamins, interact with our immune system, and interact with our nervous system. Gut-to-brain communication causes us to recognize that we are hungry and get something to eat. However, a larger amount of the brain-gut communication is subconscious, and the health of our microbiome influences our moods and the clarity of our thinking. When looking for reasons that ADD is more common than it used to be, the damage to the microbiome as a result of the increased frequency of antibiotic use, cesarean section delivery of babies (which avoids the colonization of the gut at birth), and the increase in inflammatory foods such as processed foods and fast foods are all possible contributing factors.

Physical Exercise

Many children who play a lot of video games or spend hours a day on social media on their phones are not engaging in physical exercise. Kids used to spend their days riding their bikes outside, playing with their friends, engaging in sports with the neighborhood kids. The video games preclude that type of physical exercise. Physical exercise is the best way to move blood into and through the brain, bringing necessary nutrients to the nervous tissue and keeping it healthy. Dr. Amen recommends aerobic exercise regularly for the treatment of the varied subtypes of ADD. The lack of physical exercise will negatively impact the development of the brain.

Controversies Regarding Treatment Approaches

The most common complaint regarding treatment of ADD/ADHD is the use of stimulant medications. Stimulant medications are powerful, addictive medications with many side effects. They reduce appetite, increase muscle tension (particularly in the jaw muscles), increase blood pressure, and stunt growth. They also may lose effectiveness over time.

I understand the concern regarding the overuse of stimulant medications. Prescribing stimulant medication is not a one-stop solution. Taking into account the overall health of the individual and the underlying cause of the ADD is crucial to proper treatment. Given the various subtypes of ADD/ADHD listed above it is clear that stimulant medication is not always warranted or appropriate. Patients with certain subtypes of ADD do poorly on stimulants. With the following list of herbal preparations, you will see there are alternatives. Unfortunately, as I have stated, there is nothing that works as well for increasing focus and attention as a stimulant medication. It is extremely important that when a stimulant medication is considered, the risks versus the benefits are fully explored and the subtypes of ADD/ADHD are identified and addressed. It is not in the best interest of an ADD/ADHD patient, adult or child, to be treated automatically with stimulant medications without first looking at the other possible underlying metabolic components to the illness and addressing them.

The Herbal Approach to Treating ADD

Rhodiola (*Rhodiola rosea*). Rhodiola has been well studied, especially in Russia and Sweden where it is popular. It has been shown that it is helpful for anxiety, depression, and fatigue. It is recommended to help athletes recover and to improve performance. It was used by the Vikings to improve endurance. The recommended dose is 500 mg in the morning, and you may repeat again in the afternoon. There are many commercial products in the marketplace; Jarrow and Now both offer good products.

Guido Masé, a renowned herbalist and teacher, uses high doses of rhodiola for attention deficit disorder. He recommends 4–5 grams per day of the root and 3 ml of tincture two to three times a day. It is much more practical to purchase as a tincture if you will consume it at that dose (the typical commercial supplement preparation is 500 mg per capsule). One caveat is that at high doses rhodiola can be very drying and may cause dry mouth. Guido Masé recommends taking the rhodiola along with *Ginkgo biloba*, which lowers anxiety and improves focus by improving blood flow to the brain. The calming, anti-anxiety effects balance the stimulating effect of the rhodiola.

Gingko biloba. Gingko itself is an excellent antioxidant and is well-known to increase cerebral circulation. It is also known for a calming effect. Guido Masé uses high doses of 240–480 mg of an extract standardized to 24 percent flavone glycosides. Dr. Scott Shannon, a renowned holistic pediatric psychiatrist, uses gingko to improve attention in the ADD child but finds it stimulating. He keeps the dose to 60–120 mg twice daily. There are not a lot of research studies on the effectiveness of gingko for ADD specifically, but presumably it would be working through the antioxidant process.

As an aside, Guido Masé finds that resetting the microbiome is the key to resolving ADD. He takes the roots of the disorder back to the gut. This is an interesting idea as there is some research in other fields that demonstrate the microbiome of the mother has a direct effect on the microbiome and medical conditions of her child.

Bacopa (*Bacopa monnieri*). Bacopa, also known as water hyssop, is very helpful for improving focus, attention, and brain fog from any cause. Bacopa has been well studied in the elderly population and also the child and adolescent populations; it has demonstrated improvement in focus, attention, impulsivity, and memory in all populations studied. Bacopa has also been demonstrated to have anti-anxiety effects and has proven very safe.[33, 34, 35]

The research has been done on 20 percent to 30 percent bacosides and also on 55 percent bacosides at a dose of 200–300 mg one to two times daily. However, what is available in the marketplace is 320 mg, one to two times per day. Dr. Low Dog recommends 10 percent to 20 percent bacosides, so purchase a product that is at least 20 percent bacosides for best results. Take 1 to 2 daily for twelve weeks to have a measurable effect. Bacopa is a personal favorite.

Gotu kola (*Centella asiatica*). This traditional Ayurvedic herb is commonly used for the management of anxiety and for wound healing, especially for poorly healing wounds. It appears to have the ability to stimulate nerve growth in the brain and in peripheral nerve injury. It also has been used for memory and cognitive improvement. There is literature supporting the use of gotu kola for anxiety reduction.[36] Dr. Scott Shannon (*Mental Health for the Whole Child*, p. 152) uses it for attention deficit. Gotu kola and bacopa are thought to be able to be used interchangeably and will augment one another when used simultaneously. I am fond of gotu kola and think that it works well. Organic India is a good brand. Follow the directions on the bottle. Using it with *Bacopa monnieri* is a good combination.

Dopa macuna (*Macuna puriens*). This product from Now contains 800 mg of macuna puriens and 120 mg of naturally occurring L-dopa. Recommended dosage is 1 to 2 capsules in the morning. *Macuna puriens* has been used in Ayurvedic medicine for two thousand years. It is known commonly in English as cowhage. The seeds are what is used therapeutically most often, but the root and the hairs (which cause intense itching if touched) are also sometimes used. It has widespread benefits for the body as a whole but is well known to be supportive to the nervous system.

This herb increases the amount of dopamine in the brain and was used to treat Parkinson's disease until we had L-dopa as a synthetic medication. Since ADD is improved with medications that keep the dopamine around longer, dopa macuna is helpful by increasing the amount of dopamine in the brain to begin with. Exercise caution if you are taking L-dopa for Parkinson's or any of the stimulant medications that are dopamine re-uptake inhibitors, as you can have an additive effect.[37]

Pycnogenol® (*Pinus pinaster* subsp. *Atlantica*). Pycnogenol is the product commercially made by Horphag Research from the French maritime pine. It is very well studied and is used for a wide variety of problems including ADD/ADHD. Pycnogenol is most well-known for its antioxidant effects and therefore its effects on the cardiovascular system. However, it is also widely used for the improvement of attention and focus.

Researchers have argued that ADHD is the result of a dysregulation of catecholamines (dopamine, epinephrine, and norepinephrine) resulting from oxidative stress in the brain.[38, 39] Given the strong evidence for Pycnogenol's action as an anti-oxidant it would make sense that it would be helpful for the inattentive condition caused by oxidative stress. Studies have demonstrated that Pycnogenol reduces the oxidative stress on purine (DNA) metabolism and enhances glutathione (a detoxifying chemical made in the liver) function as well as improving total antioxidant status in the children studied. The recommended dose is 100 mg daily or 1 mg per kg of body weight per day.

Useful Amino Acids

SAMe. The amino acid, S-adenosylmethione, known as SAMe, can be very stimulating to the brain and help improve mood and focus. It may be too stimulating for those who are anxious. It is contraindicated in bipolar disorder. Starting dose is 400 mg once a day, and weekly increase to a maximum of 1600 mg daily. Most people do well with 400 mg twice a day. SAMe can also be helpful for pain. It is very expensive and must be enteric coated. Buying from SAMS club or Costco discount stores is a good option.

DL-phenylalanine. The amino acid DL-phenylalanine (also known as DLPA) can be helpful for improving focus, especially if taken along with L-tyrosine. The dose for DL-phenylalanine is 750 mg daily on an empty stomach. The dose of L-tyrosine is 500 mg three times a day in between meals.

PART V

HERBAL MEDICINE FOR BIPOLAR DISORDER, SLEEP PROBLEMS, AND PAIN

· · · · · · · · · · · ·

14

BIPOLAR DISORDER

I wanted to put the chapter on bipolar disorder after the chapters on depression and anxiety because these symptom complexes are related. Bipolar disorder is a combination of depression (the depressed pole) and anxiety (the manic/hypomanic pole).

Bipolar 1 disorder is the most well-known and probably familiar to the reader. The bipolar 1 disorder is characterized by extreme mood changes between feeling good and on top of the world or highly irritable (the manic episode) and feeling deeply depressed. The episodes of mania are characterized by a period of time during which the individual has a lot of energy, is either irritable or feeling "high," with grandiosity, little need for sleep, racing thoughts, pressured speech, and poor judgment. This elevated mood can be seen as a very profound, intense anxiety. Associated with the elevated state, is insomnia, which also needs direct treatment. The opposite pole is one of a deep depression, feelings of worthlessness, hopelessness, and little energy. The bipolar depressions can be very deep and difficult to treat. The goal of treatment is to shrink the size of the mood swings so as to limit their extremes and if possible normalize the moods. These emotional states cause a great deal of anguish for both the person who is feeling them and those who love them.

The reality is that bipolar disorder is not just a swing from high to low but includes everything in between. The bipolar disorder is more of a spectrum of disorders involving a variety of mood combinations. See below for the various bipolar diagnoses that are recognized.

- ***Bipolar 1 disorder:*** Depressive episodes with one or more severe manic episodes

- ***Bipolar 2 disorder:*** Depressive episodes with one or more hypomanic episodes

- ***Cyclothymia:*** Hypomania alternating with dysthymia (unhappy mood)

- ***Cycling depressive episodes:*** Moods alternate between depression and normal, not depressed but not overly excited mood.

Over the twenty years of my practice of psychiatry, I have observed that mood swings of a variety of severity are becoming more common. Most of these mood disorders do not meet the criteria for a formal diagnosis of one of the cycling mood disorders in the DSM, but are referred to as mood disorders not otherwise specified (NOS). In a highly regarded psychiatric textbook, *Stahl's Essential Psychopharmacolgy* (third edition, published in 2008), the argument is made that 33 percent of mood disorders fall into the mood disorder NOS. I suspect today the percentage is higher. I don't have any scientific proof of why the prevalence of mood disorders NOS is increasing, but I have a suspicion it has to do with our chronic exposure to electronic stimulation of the brain.

Bipolar 1 disorder is a fairly common disorder. It often starts in the young (age 15–24) but also will show up for the first time in middle age (age 45–54). Many people live with the bipolar 1 symptoms for years before being diagnosed. There may be years during which the symptoms are in remission but then the symptoms resurface again.

A common concern of patients with bipolar disorder is whether they will pass it on to their children. Unfortunately, it is not an easy question to answer. Bipolar disorder is an inherited disorder with a 5 percent to 10 percent risk in first-degree relatives but it does not follow a predictable pattern of inheritance. We cannot say whether the disorder will be passed on and to whom. The disorder may be present in each generation or skip several generations. We just cannot tell.

Bipolar disorder is often associated with other physical illnesses. It seems to be associated with irritable bowel syndrome and asthma. The inflammatory process and the physiological relationships between organ systems (gut-brain and lung-brain) seem to be responsible for these associations. There is also an association of anxiety and attention deficit disorders in bipolar disorder.

Lifestyle treatments can make a difference in the severity of bipolar disorder and the type and amount of medication needed to stabilize moods. What is clear from the relationship to inflammation is that a focus on anti-inflammatory lifestyle and diet can be of great value. Bipolar disorder may be a progressive disorder with increasing episodes of mania and a greater resistance to treatment, so optimizing treatment early is imperative.

The purpose of treatment for a bipolar patient is to stabilize the moods so the ups and downs become smaller, more manageable, and less frequent. The mainstay of conventional medical treatment is a mood stabilizer medication. See below for a list of medications commonly used. All these medications have side effects, and the risk and benefit must be fully discussed with the patient. The anti-psychotic medications are most helpful in those whose manic or depressive episodes become psychotic. They are helpful in stopping the mania and also in preventing recurring mania.

Common Bipolar Medications

Lithium	Considered the gold standard	Mineral, has effects on the kidney and the thyroid, needs close monitoring of blood levels.
Carbamazepine	Tegretol	Has some sedating side effects and needs close monitoring of blood levels.
Valproic acid	Depakote/Depakene	Weight gain and sedation are common and needs close monitoring of blood levels and liver function.
Lamotrigine	Lamictal, not FDA approved	Commonly used and effective. Well tolerated. No blood levels needed.
Oxcarbazepine	Trileptal, not FDA approved	Break-down product of carbamazepine. Well tolerated, no blood levels needed. Moderately effective.
Topiramate	Topamax, not FDA approved	Not effective for mood stabilization.

Common Anti-Psychotic Medications for Bipolar Disorder

Aripriprazole	Abilify, FDA approved as a first line treatment	Available in oral and monthly injectable forms.
Cariprazine	Vraylar	Effective but very expensive.
Lurasidone	Latuda, FDA approved for the depressive component of the bipolar cycle	Moderately effective but also expensive.
Asenapine	Saphris	Highly sedating, dissolvable tab.
Olanzapine	Zyprexa	Commonly used in hospitals. Significant increase in weight gain and sedation. Often used for sleep.
Risperidone	Risperdal	Commonly used in hospitals.
Ziprasidone	Geodon	Less weight gain and less sedation. Must be taken with food.

Mania poses serious consequences in life. There is poor judgment, so there can be inappropriate financial decisions, sexual improprieties, impulsive and irresponsible behavior. One patient filled his pickup truck with over two hundred teddy bears. One woman purchased one hundred tubes of the same lipstick. Impulsive behaviors can include the sudden quitting of a job, moving to another town, the abandonment of a family. There can be hyper-sexuality with increased sexual activity but no judgment as to the person with whom the sex takes place. As you can imagine, these impulsive episodes of poor judgment can cause a great deal of harm to the individual and their loved ones.

The depressive episodes can be very severe and difficult to treat. There is great suffering and a high risk of suicide.

As mentioned above, there are many examples of cycling in moods that do not meet the criteria of bipolar disorder or its variants. I find these patients can improve with mood stabilizers even though the diagnosis of bipolar disorder is not officially made.

The reader will notice that so far there has not been a mention of herbs for the treatment of bipolar disorder. The reason for that is there are no herbs specific for bipolar disorder. The herbs are chosen based on the individual characteristics of the person with the disorder and the type of symptoms that they demonstrate. As explained above, there are many variants of bipolar disorder and also of mood cycling in general. The focus of treatment is on improving the symptoms.

The first approach to the stabilization of bipolar disorder is to focus on the foundational components of health: diet, sleep, exercise, stress reduction, good relationships with others. The diet needs to be whole foods, nothing processed, avoiding the seed oils such as canola oil, soybean oil, palm kernel oil, and corn oil. Most whole foods require preparation at home but there are some shortcuts. You can purchase a roasted whole chicken from the grocery store and have a whole food that is precooked but not processed. You can purchase a box of mixed greens that are fresh and not processed. Now there are also companies that deliver whole foods to your door. Companies like www.territoryfoods.com; www.trifectanutrition.com; www.greenchef.com will bring whole foods to you.

Eating something that is frozen, preserved, or highly processed has markedly lessened flavor and often contains preservatives that are harmful to health. The best foods for health are those that are prepared at home. Think about food as providing the building blocks of your neurotransmitters. The healthier the building blocks, the healthier the neurotransmitters.

Sleep is important for all of us, but particularly important for the bipolar patient. When there is consistent insomnia it often is a precursor to a manic episode. There are many natural approaches to improving sleep that will be discussed in the next chapter. Sleep is the time the brain washes itself and the time when repair takes place. The brain needs this down time just like any other organ in the body. Good quality sleep is what makes us feel rejuvenated and ready to move forward with the day.

Exercise is very important for the management of any mental illness. Aerobic exercise is the best way to encourage blood flow to the brain, but it is not always possible—especially if one is in the depressed phase of the disorder. I also like to reframe exercise as movement. Moving the body in the form of dancing, walking, tai chi, yoga—anything that you enjoy—even a little bit can be very helpful. Also, for some, doing movement in a class or group is helpful. For those who do not want to leave the house there are YouTube videos of tai chi and yoga that you can do in the comfort and safety of your own home. Moving the body gets your energy moving. Depression is a state when your energy is quiet and heavy. Moving that energy loosens the heaviness and improves and lightens the mood. Be aware that during a manic phase, the exercise can become excessive and we must be careful to avoid injury.

Stress reduction is very important. There are many techniques such as meditation, deep breathing, and relaxation techniques. Picking one that helps you and that you can relate to is the only way to be successful. Stress has a profound effect on overall health and on the health and function of the brain specifically. Stress will raise the level of inflammation in the brain dramatically and will limit your ability to heal.

Another perspective on stress is overwork or doing too much. Sometimes we have to come to an acceptance that the lifestyle we have chosen is hurting us. Maybe we want to work as hard as we possibly can for financial reasons, but there is also a high price to be paid for that. Maybe we need less work and a simpler lifestyle. Maybe we have to leave a toxic relationship or give up something else. If you feel your stress level is too high, examine your lifestyle. See if there is something that you can simplify or a relationship that is too distressing. Do the best you can to lessen what is realistically possible to lessen.

Having good relationships with others is another component that is very important. Often the bipolar patient has damaged relationships because of erratic behavior. Using counseling to help establish a social network of support can be very helpful. The bipolar patient should not feel alone.

Another aspect of bipolar disorder is the toxic effect of substance abuse. Substance abuse can cause harm to any brain. Depending on the substance and the amount of abuse, the effects can be devastating. What I see over and over is that substance abuse, including smoking marijuana and drinking alcohol, are destabilizing to the bipolar brain. I had a conversation with a young man with bipolar disorder recently who on his own came to realize that every time he smoked marijuana it caused his mood to be unstable the next day. He had to stop smoking marijuana for a period of two months before he had that epiphany. Usually a point of contrast is necessary. There are some patients who have manic episodes only after smoking marijuana. For this reason, I require complete sobriety from all substances if I am to try to stabilize the bipolar patient with minimal medication.

The use of herbal medicine for bipolar disorder can be very helpful if used judiciously. If there is psychosis or suicidality then medications are warranted. In my experience, medications are always needed when there is psychosis. The herbals can be used in conjunction with the medication to keep the medication dose low and thereby limit possible side effects. Working with a qualified medical practitioner is absolutely necessary.

All the herbs listed in the anxiety section and the depression section can be used to improve the moods that occur in the bipolar patient. I have yet to find an herbal remedy or remedies that improves the swinging between poles.

Using herbals that are nourishing to the nervous system is valuable. These include the adaptogens and the nootropics (previously called nervines or tonics).

There are a couple of herbs that deserve special mention.

An adaptogen that I use frequently is ashwagandha (*Withania somnifera*). Because there is so much involvement of the HPA axis in all mental disorders, ashwagandha is a go-to for stabilization. It is one of the most calming of the herbs we have and can help sleep be restorative. Ashwagandha has been used to restore health due to illness, extreme stress, and nervous exhaustion. In the Western world, most ashwagandha is consumed in the form of tea, tincture, or extract in a pill. However, in Ayurvedic medicine many medicinals are administered as an enema. Ashwagandha in high dose can be used to manage a manic episode when administered as an enema. To make the enema, mix 1 tablespoon of ashwagandha herb (cut and sifted) to 10 ounces of water. Simmer for 5 minutes and cool. Strain. Hold in the rectum for 30 minutes if possible. The patient may need to use daily for up to five days in a row. It is best used at the beginning of a manic episode to prevent it from developing or to nip it in the bud. Most Westerners are not open to the idea of rectal administration of medication but for one who might be it is an interesting treatment modality.

A particular concept that applies to many mental illnesses but particularly to the bipolar patient is to support and tonify as well as calm. The depressive phase often needs cortisol support and the manic phase often needs calming. Creating a combination of support and calming can be very useful.

To support the energy of the body and mind, licorice can be helpful. The licorice root (*Glycyrrhiza glabra*) is supportive of the adrenal system. The licorice will inhibit the enzyme that breaks down the cortisol the adrenals make and therefore give more support to the brain and body. With more cortisol the body can manage stress more effectively. It is beneficial to reduce the anxiety at the same time as you support the adrenal system. One product that works well is Metagenics Licorice Plus. It contains licorice root to slow the breakdown of cortisol, allowing the body to have the cortisol around longer. Having the cortisol around longer helps the body manage stress better. It also has an herb called Rhemannia glutinosa which helps support the kidney. In Chinese medicine the kidney is the source of life, and supporting the kidney can be calming and stabilizing.

For those who also suffer from attention deficits, *Bacopa monnieri* and gotu kola (*Centella asiatica*) are useful to improve focus and simultaneously reduce anxiety. These two herbs are used interchangeably in Ayurvedic medicine and I think about them together as though they are one herb. *Bacopa monnieri* is currently being studied for memory improvement.

Pycnogenol has excellent antioxidant effects and has been shown to improve focus. The amino acid L-theanine is also a great asset as it reduces anxiety by increasing GABA and simultaneously increases dopamine which improves focus. L-theanine can be used as a standard dose, regularly taken three times a day or as needed before an anxiety-producing event such as a date or a job interview.

How an Herbalist Treats Bipolar Disorder

Lou is a fifty-four-year-old male, married with three adult children. He has been manic most of his life, commonly working twenty hours a day. He was sharp, able to analyze complex information quickly and write clearly about it. But lately, he's been having trouble with memory, concentration, and his ability to write. His mother died four years ago, which affected him deeply and he fell into a deep depression. Not long after, he was diagnosed with bipolar disorder. At the time he presented to our clinic he was deeply depressed but came to us for his cognitive impairment.

Lou's cognitive impairment started a year prior to presenting at our clinic. Along with the memory problems, he had an increase in his ADHD symptoms, having great difficulty staying on a task and had a great deal of difficulty completing any task, however minor. His primary care physician placed him on short-term disability due to cognitive decline. He was assessed for a sleeping disorder to rule out sleep apnea, a common cause for memory impairment. He was given no other diagnosis or treatment.

His significant medical issues include type 2 diabetes mellitus, being overweight, chronic irritable bowel disorder, diarrhea type. He had diarrhea daily and frequently throughout the day. He has also had difficulty sleeping and often took Benadryl to put himself to sleep.

The treatment for improving memory requires a resolution of all the metabolic factors that insult the brain and cause inflammation leading to the development of amyloid plaques. The plaques are the result of these metabolic insults. In Lou's case, the brain insults included poor gastrointestinal health (chronic diarrhea and irritable bowel disease), insulin resistance, type 2 diabetes, obesity, high stress level, poor sleep, anti-cholinergic medications (choline is what forms our memories, anti-cholinergics make memory difficult), and bipolar disorder, which was not stable.

In order to address the underlying metabolic issues we first had to stabilize the mood swings and work on his lifestyle. He was taking lithium when he came to me but at his request, because another family member with bipolar disorder did well on carbamazepine, we started him on carbamazepine for mood stability.

To improve the memory we started with diet. He was placed on an elimination diet to resolve the chronic diarrhea. The diarrhea was preventing the absorption of his medications and supplements as they were passing directly through him undigested. He discovered he had an allergy to nuts, soy, and eggs, and when he avoided these foods the diarrhea stopped. He also had an endoscopy that revealed Barrett's esophagus (a precancerous lesion) and was placed on a proton pump inhibitor.

We also thought there was an anxiety component to the diarrhea, and I recommended chamomile and skullcap tea. He could make it as a tea and sip it throughout the day to keep him calm. This would also improve the stress level and improve his quality of sleep. Chamomile is a good herb for digestive health and is also a mild calmative.

Once the diarrhea was resolved we moved on to the keto diet. The keto diet has excellent research behind it as being able to improve cognitive impairment. He took to the keto diet readily and implemented it easily. He lost weight and with the addition of berberine supplementation he was able to get off his diabetes medications. This was done in concert with his primary care physician. I also encouraged him to eat organic foods and avoid processed foods.

He had periods of being compliant with the diet and periods of time when he would binge eat. When he binged his diarrhea and diabetes returned. He had to be restarted on the metformin and I encouraged him to take vitamin B12 along with it as metformin blocks B12 absorption as does the proton pump inhibitor.

He was also encouraged to do twenty minutes of aerobic activity daily.

Additional supplementation that was recommended was 3000 mg daily of the fatty acids found in fish oil, and to help him sleep we added skullcap throughout the day. We also had him take the nootropic Brain and Memory Power Boost available through www.brainmd.com.

The biggest challenge for him was the mood stability. When something upsetting happened in his life he would run off and eat. Binging behavior, whether it is drinking alcohol or eating excessively, is common during a manic phase of bipolar disorder. He eventually decided to attend an inpatient program followed by an outpatient program for eating disorders. He found great benefit at the inpatient program and his eating behavior has improved.

15

HERBAL MEDICINE FOR SLEEP

Having a good night's sleep makes the world seem like a better place. We have all had the experience of not sleeping well at some point in our lives. We know from experience that we are less alert, think less clearly and quickly, become more irritable, and make more mistakes. Sleep is critical to our health and mental function.

Research has shown that there is a bell curve for the need for sleep. Most adults fall in the seven to nine hours of sleep requirement. Children and teenagers need much more sleep. We need less sleep as we age.

Our sleep can be disrupted and disturbed by any number of things. If we have something on our mind—a fight with a spouse, a child or work challenges—sleep will be disrupted. This is a normal experience, and as long as it does not become a daily experience to rise to the level of a disorder, normal sleep patterns should return once the challenge is resolved.

Disrupted and poor sleep is associated with many chronic medical illnesses such as increased risk of obesity, type 2 diabetes mellitus and insulin resistance, as well as depression. (See chapter 10 on insulin resistance and its effect on cognition and mood.) When sleep is chronically disrupted there is a profound effect on the rest of the body. The endocrine system, the autonomic nervous system (fight or flight system), and the immune system all become dysregulated, leaving us vulnerable to infection and illness.

Psychiatric disorders commonly cause sleep disturbances. Anxiety is one of the most common reasons that one is unable to fall asleep or stay asleep. The anxious brain is a busy brain at night, thinking constantly, sometimes about unimportant things, but it just won't stop thinking and that prevents you from falling asleep. The anxious brain may be working even while asleep. It will wake you at 2, 3, or 4 A.M. and immediately start being busy again so you cannot go back to sleep easily. The anxiety can make your sleep fitful, causing you to toss and turn all night. This can keep you from feeling rested even if you sleep through the night or get a full eight hours of time in bed.

One characteristic of anxiety is the fear of losing control or feeling as though you are giving up control. This can be an important component of the inability to fall asleep. If letting your mind relax is equated with a loss of control, it can be a terrifying experience to go to sleep. The fear of loss of control is best treated with therapy, cognitive behavioral therapy in particular, can be very helpful. Often, what helps with the ability to fall asleep at night is to relax during the day and lower the threshold of anxiety so there is a shorter distance to fall when trying to get to sleep. The best treatment for anxiety-disrupted sleep of course, is to treat the anxiety. (See chapter 12 and the treatments that follow.)

One important component of falling asleep is feeling safe. What makes someone feel safe varies widely from person to person. For some, a large dog and extra locks on the door may help.

For others, using a white noise machine or leaving their phone on their bedside table "in case of emergency" may help. (I usually recommend leaving your cell phone out of the bedroom, but if a phone nearby is comforting you may choose to leave it. I would suggest powering it off and putting it in a drawer if possible, so you're less likely to scroll through it at bedtime.) Many people who are survivors of sexual abuse associate the abuse with the night and with the bed. Therefore, it can be very difficult to relax enough to fall asleep; the hypervigilance will keep the person awake. Doing whatever it takes to help you feel safe in your own bedroom is a priority in improving sleep and restfulness.

Depression is also a cause of disrupted sleep. Depression often causes the normal circadian rhythm of sleep to reverse. For example, it is normal to sleep in the nighttime and be awake in the daytime. Our bodies respond to natural light rhythms and melatonin helps keep those rhythms in proper order. When a person is depressed, they will sleep during the day and be awake at night. A depressed mood may keep you asleep for hours of the day, or at least in bed, not wanting to do anything. Here you may deal with hypersomnia, defined as excessive sleeping and daytime sleepiness. This is a natural consequence of the depressed state of mind, but it also will make it very difficult to treat the depression itself. Therefore, it is very important to improve the sleep of the depressed person. I highly recommend trying to stay awake during the day as many hours as possible and out of the bed if even just to the couch. Also, mild exercise—even just a walk around the block—can make a world of difference. Dr. Zach Bush has a simple four-minute exercise routine that moves blood, gets nitric oxide moving, and can get your blood flowing without anything strenuous, and anyone can do it as long as they can stand up and move their arms. You can find a video explaining this workout at www.youtube.com/watch?v=PwJCJToQmps. To ask a depressed person to exercise is often met with great resistance. The last thing anyone wants to do when depressed is to exercise. I understand that. So, do not think about it as exercise, but rather as movement. Just moving the body, not allowing yourself to be horizontal in bed for hours on end, can begin to shift the weight of depression. The four-minute exercise routine can be very helpful, even if you do not make it past one repetition.

A note about night owls. There are some people who naturally prefer to be awake during the night and asleep during the day. I am glad for those people because we need them in our society. They are the guards that stand watch at night without falling sleep, and the doctors and nurses that take the night shift. However, when night owls get depressed, working night shift does not do them any favors. It is always better to try to be asleep before midnight when treating a depressed state of mind.

The depressed person may also have early morning awakening, waking at 2, 3, or 4 A.M. There may be some anxiety mixed in with the depressed mood and both depression and anxiety may need to be addressed.

The best way to treat the hypersomnia, insomnia and early morning awakening is to treat the depressed mood. (See chapter 3.)

The patient with bipolar disorder particularly needs to have good sleep. Insomnia is often an early symptom that signals the onset of a manic episode. When the mood is stable the sleep is usually stable, meaning the person can fall asleep and stay asleep and feel sufficiently rested the next day. During a manic episode, the nervous system has so much energy that to quiet it down may require heroic efforts. It can be very impressive how revved up the nervous system can actually become. For this reason, it is a good idea to try to nip it in the bud and make sure there is sleep every night, preferably with a bedtime before midnight. Once you let the circadian rhythm get out of control, it is much harder to control the mood swings.

I had one patient who would not sleep for days in a row. She did not have bipolar disorder in the sense of mood swings, nor did she have depression or anxiety in the conventional manner. She had a history of alcoholism. What was striking to me was that her insomnia cycled as though she had bipolar 2 disorder with the insomnia as the only manifestation of the mania. She would be miserable and would come into the hospital so she could get medication to help her sleep. The only thing that made a difference for her sleep was a shot of an antipsychotic medication. She was eventually placed on a monthly injection which stabilized her cyclic insomnia. She was not hospitalized again after that.

Sleep apnea is a special case of disrupted sleep. I have seen sleep apnea in the overweight person and in the normal weight person. If someone is having trouble with being excessively tired in the daytime, falling asleep at traffic lights, even though they "sleep" eight hours a night, it is worth a sleep study. Sleep apnea is a major medical hazard, not only to mental health but to overall health. It contributes to high blood pressure, vascular disease, and mental illness. Many people do not want to do a sleep study because they do not think they will be able to sleep in such an artificial and highly tested environment and fear there will be a false result. Many also will not go for testing because they do not want to wear the face mask required to treat the sleep apnea. Luckily, there are newer methods of evaluation and treatment being developed. Sleep apnea has to be treated to get a handle on the underlying psychiatric disorders.

I am not a fan of medication for sleep. There are many side effects, there may be addiction, and there is failure. The medication often "poops out" and the dosage needs to be raised, or the medication type or class needs to be changed. If it is possible to improve sleep without medication, I prefer it. Sometimes, like the case described above, it is necessary to use medication. Also, with judicious use, medication and herbals may be safely used together, allowing the dose of medication to be low.

Avoid over-the-counter products that contain diphenhydramine, commercially known as Benadryl. This chemical is an anticholinergic medication, the side effect of which is sedation. Choline is needed for the creation of memory and a chemical that is anti-choline is anti-memory formation. Other side effects include weight gain (it also makes you hungry), dry mouth, and dry gut, which may lead to constipation. The diphenhydramine products are particularly harmful to the elderly.

Using Herbal Medicine for Improved Sleep

Important Note: As always, if you have significant sleep issues, consult your health care practitioner. All the recommendations below do not take the place of good sleep habits.

Anxiety is a common reason people have difficulty sleeping. All the herbs in the chapter on anxiety apply here. Lowering daytime anxiety is often the key to a good night's sleep; it will help you fall asleep more easily and also allow you to stay asleep.

Helpful Amino Acids

Melatonin. Melatonin is a popular sleep aid. It is a hormone with many functions, including the synchronization of biological rhythms; the two most important are the circadian rhythm (which controls the hormonal system) and the normal need for sleep. It is effective in inducing sleep in only 25 percent to 30 percent of the population and its effect is dose dependent; the higher the dose the more likely it will be to make you sleep. It is often used in combination with many other supplements and products that do help with sleep. There are a few side effects of melatonin that are not well known. One is that if the dose is too high you will awaken with a startle. If this happens to you, reduce the dose. Some people complain of a morning hangover, so reduce the dose if this happens to you.

Melatonin reduces the sleep latency time, the time it takes you to fall asleep, so it may be helpful if you have trouble falling asleep. It does not particularly help with staying asleep. If you have both problems, consider an extended release melatonin preparation or a combination product.

L-theanine. An amino acid derived from the leaf of a green tea, L-theanine stimulates the GABA receptor to quiet the thinking so you can fall asleep. There are some commercial preparations sold widely over the counter, even at the local drug store, that contain both theanine and melatonin. This is a very nice combination.

If you want to try it alone, start with 100 mg at bedtime and go up from there. After you take the first dose, if you are still awake forty-five minutes later, take another dose and so on until you find the dose you need. Do this on a night before a day when you do not have to get up at a particular time or have a lot of responsibility. Taking the doses throughout the night is likely to give you a bit of a hangover. Once you have established the necessary milligrams needed you should not have the hangover.

Tryptophan and 5-htp. These two amino acids are the precursors to serotonin and can be very relaxing. They are useful for relaxation, mood enhancement, anxiety reduction, and sleep. They are particularly helpful for *keeping* one asleep, probably due to their anti-anxiety effects. *Do not take them together*; try one or the other.

The dose for tryptophan is 500 mg at bedtime for a week, increasing by 500 mg nightly until the desired effect is achieved or the maximum dose of 1500 mg is reached. The dose for 5-htp is 100 mg at bedtime for a week, increasing by 100 mg weekly to a maximum of 300 mg daily. You may split the doses during the day as daytime relaxation is often helpful for a good night's sleep.

Commercial Preparations for Mild Insomnia

Put Me To Sleep Naturally. This is a preparation developed by Dr. Amen that many of my patients swear by. It is worth a try if your sleep disturbance is due to tension and stress. This product contains: melatonin 1.25 mg, GABA 300 mg, *Magnesium glycinate*/malate 100 mg, vitamin B6 10 mg (a calming vitamin), 5-htp 50 mg, and L-theanine 100 mg. The work horse of this product is the melatonin which is supported by the remaining ingredients. Available on www.brainmd.com. Follow the directions on the bottle.

Sound sleep. This product is sold by GAIA herbs and is a nice combination of sleep enhancing herbs. It is helpful for mild or occasional insomnia. This product contains passionflower (*Passiflora incarnata*), American skullcap (*Scutellaria lateriflora*), kava (*Piper methysticum*), valerian (*Valeriana officinalis*), California poppy (*Eschscholzia californica*), and hops (*Humulus lupulus*). Follow the directions on the bottle.

Herbal Preparations

A note about herbal preparations: I am listing many possible options and some of their specific characteristics. You can try each one and see if any one herb works for you. Usually, they work best as a combination allowing synergistic activity among the herbs. Therefore, you will see some combinations listed as well along with references.

Sleep Disturbances Due to Anxiety or Busy Brain

Phosphatidylserine. This amino acid is helpful if you awaken in the morning with intense anxiety. Take it before you go to bed so your morning is relaxed. This is sold over the counter by the name PS100. Follow the directions on the product that you buy.

Chinese polygala (*Polygala tenuifolia, Yuan zhi*). This herb is traditionally used for anxiety and fear. It is sedating in nature, so it is able to help with sleep. It can be particularly helpful for those whose sleep is difficult to come by because of fear of falling asleep or not feeling safe. It seems to be helpful for improving cognition. Large doses can cause nausea and vomiting. Do not use with gastritis, ulcers, or pregnancy. It is available as granules (that are made into a tea when steeped in hot water) and tinctures. Do not confuse it with Senega snakeroot (*Polygala senega*). Follow directions on the bottle of the product that you purchase. Hawaii Pharm is a good brand.

Fu shen (*Poria cocos/spirit*). This is a lesser known medicinal mushroom whose mycelia form a solid ball underground that resembles a coconut which can be quite large. The ball is harvested and made into a tincture. Fu ling is another name for the mushroom, but I have not seen this name sold commercially. Fu ling pi is sold commercially and is the skin of the mushroom used as a diuretic. Fu shen is the inner white strands of the mushroom which is used for insomnia and is very uplifting to the spirit, so it may also be used for depression. It is available as an alcohol-free tincture from Hawaii Pharm. Follow the directions on the bottle of the preparation that you purchase. Please be aware that it is very sedating so try it first at night, preferably before a day when you have few responsibilities. If you feel a hangover the next day, reduce the dose. I personally have used this product and find it to be very sedating, and the next day I feel happy and nothing bothers me.

Nutmeg (*Myristica fragrans*). Nutmeg is best known as a spice used in cooking. It is also helpful for sleep. It is best used fresh, but if you do not have a whole nutmeg you can try the dried powder available in the grocery store. Start with a quarter of a teaspoon in any medium you prefer (oatmeal, cottage cheese, tea, etc.). Take one hour before sleep. Increase the dose by ¼ teaspoon every three days until you reach ¾ teaspoon or you are sleeping like a baby. My experience is that nutmeg provides a very deep sleep. Be cautious with the dose, anything over ¾ teaspoon may cause hallucinations. Simply purchase the whole nutmeg from the grocery store and grate it fresh at home.

Hops (*Humulus lupulus*). Hops is most well-known for beer, but it is also a relaxant. It helps relax muscle spasm and also calms the mind for sleep. It is often mixed with other herbs (valerian and lemon balm) to help with sleep. Easley and Horne describe it as "best on hot, damp people who are often over-weight and red-faced with fiery personalities and have poor digestion and insomnia" (*The Modern Herbal Dispensatory*, p. 247). Take 2 dropperfuls at bedtime to improve sleep. My go-to for alcohol-free tincture is Hawaii Pharm. Some find the alcohol tinctures to be more potent. Follow the directions on the product that you purchase.

Linden flowers (*Tilia europea*). Sold in Europe as a beverage and consumed much like Americans drink tea or coffee. It is used for its relaxing quality and mild, sedative effects. It is helpful for reducing the effects of stress and tension. Drink a cup one to three times a day. It has a pleasant flavor. Also available as a tincture. Linden flowers is safe for children. It can also be used in a bath for relaxation. Place an ounce (⅔ of a cup) of herb in a cheesecloth and put in a bath or make a strong tea (defined as steeping for 10–15 minutes) and add to the bath. It is very relaxing taken this way. I recommend trying the bath on a night before a day you have no responsibilities.

Wild oats (*Avena fatua, A. sativa*). This plant is a nerve support that is specific for exhaustion due to depression. It may also be helpful for withdrawal from addictions. The tincture needs to be made from fresh milky seed of the herb. Wild oats

193

are very helpful for wound up children that are hyperactive due to anxiety. Make the tea and the child can drink it freely. An alcohol-free extract can also be mixed in a juice. In the United States, most products are sold as *Avena sativa*. Herb Pharm carries an alcohol-free tincture. Not for use in pregnancy.

Passionflower (*Passiflora incarnata*). This beautiful flower reduces muscle tension and relieves a busy brain. It is most helpful for quieting the mind to allow you to fall asleep. It will tend to wear off during the night and for that reason is often mixed with other herbs such as valerian (*Valeriana officinalis*) or skullcap (*Scutellaria lateriflora*). Available as a tincture and in supplement form. It is also a pleasant tasting tea if you prefer. Follow the directions on the product that you purchase.

Catnip (*Nepeta cataria*). Not just for cats, catnip is a mild relaxant and calmative. This plant is helpful for young children, even infants. Serve as a tea. Never boil the herb, but rather steep it. It is very effective for calming fussy babies and children when combined with fennel. Take 1 cup of tea two to three times a day. Easley and Horne describe catnip as useful for irritable bowel syndrome due to stress. It is an excellent anti-spasmodic for the colon when made with fresh leaf tincture. Easley and Horne prefer a fresh leaf glycerite of 90 percent glycerin (the standard is 70 percent). Take 1–2 teaspoons up to three times daily. Available as a tea, as the herb, and as a glycerite.

To Improve Sleep Interfered with by Pain

California poppy (*Eschscholzia californica*). This herb is useful when pain is the reason that sleep is disturbed. As a member of the poppy family, it has mild pain-relieving properties. It is also sedating. California poppy will give you a positive opiate test so be aware of that if you get drug tested at your job. It is also sold as an alcohol-free tincture combined with valerian. Follow the directions on the product that you purchase.

Valerian (*Valeriana oficinalis*). Valerian is probably the most widely sold over-the-counter sleep aid in Europe. It is also an anti-spasmodic and will improve muscle relaxation. It is often combined with other herbal remedies. Research has shown that it takes several weeks for the valerian alone to be effective for reducing the sleep latency time. Therefore, it is combined with other herbs which work more quickly and over time the valerian will support better sleep. The limiting aspect of valerian is the smell. It has a strong musky scent described as dirty socks. There are some who do not mind the smell and you should consider that when trying this product as you may be one who does not mind it. Valerian is a good anti-anxiety herb and if the reason you are not sleeping well is that you have anxiety in the form of busy thinking keeping you from falling asleep or waking frequently during the night, it is a good choice. Occasionally there are people for whom valerian acts as a stimulant and may worsen insomnia. There is no way to know if this is you until you try it. Because it has a strong anti-anxiety effect it may worsen depression. It is available in capsule and tincture form. Follow the directions on the bottle of the product you purchase.

Jamaican dogwood (*Piscidia erythrina/piscipula*). Jamaican dogwood is a potent sedative and also has pain-relieving properties, especially for nerve pain. It is known as fish poison tree because it is poisonous to fish. It is *not* poisonous to people (unless you are a mermaid). It is, however, a potent sedative. It is useful for those who have difficulty sleeping because of pain. It is available as an alcohol-free tincture from Hawaii Pharm and as a supplement from Secrets of the Tribe. Follow the directions on the bottle of the product you purchase.

Wild lettuce (*Lactuca virosa*). This is a lesser-known plant used for its relaxant and analgesic properties. The herbal tea is bitter and is best combined with other herbs or taken as a supplement. Wild lettuce is used to relieve pain and to impart relaxation to both the mind and the body. It is helpful for improving sleep disturbed by anxiety and worry or pain in the body. It is commercially available as an alcohol-free extract from Hawaii Pharm. Take one to two dropperfuls at bedtime. Also available in capsule form.

For General Support of the Nervous System

There are numerous herbs that support the nervous system. Following here are a few that are particularly helpful for sleep.

Ashwagandha (*Withania somnifera*). As the word somnifera (somni = sleep + fer = going) would indicate this herb encourages sleep. What I have observed with it is that the sleep is more restful rather than an immediate feeling of sleepiness. Gaia herbs makes a good product. Take twice daily.

Skullcap (*Scutellaria lateriflora*). Known for relaxing qualities, skullcap is a favorite of mine. This is an excellent nootropic, tonic herb that relaxes nervousness. It is often combined with passionflower. Taken throughout the day it will relieve much nervousness and tension to allow for an easier time falling asleep.

Eleuthero (*Eleuthero senticosus*). Formerly known as Siberian ginseng, it normalizes the HPA axis and is useful for those who do not sleep well. It is an herb that is appropriate for long-term use. It is good to use for those who gorge on carbs, especially when anxious (think nighttime bingeing). It is best used for those who work hard, play hard and hardly sleep. Available as the actual herb, herb powder, tincture, or supplement pill. Follow the directions on the bottle of the product you purchase.

Dr. Jill Stansbury, a renowned naturopathic physician, recommends herbs that increase circulation for the elderly rather than using sedative herbs. The elderly are often more sensitive to sedation and often have decreased circulation to the brain. I think she makes a very good point. She recommends supporting the circulation with the following herbs: *Panax ginseng, Gingko biloba,* and *Withania somnifera.*

General Herbal Sedative Combination

Ashwagandha (*Withania somnifera*)

Oats (*Avena sativa*)

Passionflower (*Passiflora incarnata*)

Valerian (*Valeriana officinalis*)

Purchase the above as tinctures or non-alcohol glycerites. Mix together in equal parts and take 1–2 dropperfuls an hour before bed and again at bedtime.

Herbal Formularies for Health Professionals, Volume 4, Neurology, Psychiatry and Pain Management, Dr. Jill Stansbury N.D. (Chelsea Green Publishing, 2020)

Good Sleep Hygiene (Habits)

Good sleep hygiene has been shown to improve the quality of sleep and the subjective experience of restfulness. Practice the following sleep habits:

- Sleep in a cool, dark room. Use blackout curtains if needed.
- Keep the room quiet and undisturbed.
- Remove pets from the bedroom if you feel they may be disturbing your sleep cycle.
- Go to sleep at the same time every night and get up at the same time every morning even if on vacation or a weekend.
- Stop screen exposure two hours prior to sleep.
- Move the phone and other electronics out of the bedroom.
- Remove the television from the bedroom.
- Use the bed only for sleep and sex, not to work, especially on the computer.
- Start your bedtime routine, brushing teeth, washing face, changing into pajamas early, so that you don't wake yourself up doing these things just before lying down to sleep.
- Avoid alcohol before bed; it is initially a relaxant and then it becomes a stimulant and disrupts the quality of sleep.
- Try to avoid naps.

- Take a bath. Two hours before bed can be helpful. There are excellent essential oils that can help relax you. Try two drops each of lavender, Roman chamomile, black pepper, and rosemary. You may also add in some Epsom salts or a strong tea of relaxing herb such as linden flowers, also known as *Tilia*.

- Exercise. Exercising during the day can also be helpful to lower the tension level at night. Exercising at night can help relax some people but can also wake you up. Listen to your body to know which is right for you.

- Do not eat for three hours prior to bedtime.

- Never watch the clock. If you find yourself wanting to know how long you have been awake, get out of bed and do something boring. No screens!

Nighttime Rituals That Help with Sleep

Evening baths. Baths are known in medicine as hydrotherapy. They have been used for centuries as a treatment tool for relaxation, improving circulation, and in ancient times were utilized frequently and for many ailments. Images of Roman, Greek, and Egyptian baths are easy to find in any history book. Hippocrates recommended hydrotherapy for many illnesses. Many people travel to natural springs which have a high mineral content as well as high heat.

Most of the hydrotherapy in ancient times was used with essential oils and herbs. I think that is a great idea for modern day treatment of anxiety, tension, and insomnia. Below are some suggestions of herbs and essential oils that may be of value in helping you relax enough to sleep.

Take a warm bath for at least twenty minutes before going to bed. Let your body soak in the tub with relaxing herbs and or oils and soft lighting. It should be a comfortable experience. To add the herbs to the bath, place them in a cheesecloth bag and place in the water as you run the bath. Let the herbs steep into the bathwater. You can also make a strong tea by infusing the herbs in water that has just stopped boiling and let the tea steep for 10–15 minutes. You can also make a decoction (simmer the herbs for 20 minutes), strain and cool. Add the tea or decoction to the bath water. You may try one of these herbs or mix several of them together. Try various combinations to find which one works the best for you. Be sure to stay well hydrated.

Relaxing Herbs for the Bath

- Linden flowers (*Tilia europaea*)
- Chamomile (*Matricaria chamomilla*)
- Kava kava (*Piper methysticum*), very good for relaxing muscles
- Lavender (*Lavandula*)
- Catnip (*Napeta cataria*)
- Rosemary (*Salvia rosmarinus*), also helpful for muscle relaxation and clarity of thinking
- Hops (*Humulus lupulus*)

Relaxing Essential Oils for the Bath

(Use 1–3 drops of a single oil per bath, total of 6 drops per bath if combining oils.)

- Lavender
- Roman chamomile
- Black pepper (very good for muscle relaxation)
- Rosemary

A note of safety when using essential oils: Avoid using citrus oils directly in the bath as they may burn the skin. You can add a carrier oil such as coconut oil or a little soap to allow the oils to mix better in the bath as essential oils are not soluble in water.

Physical Medicine and Mind/Body Therapies That Can Help with Sleep

Acupuncture can be very helpful. Acupuncture can give you an overall balance but there are also specific points helpful for sleep. The acupuncturist may offer some Chinese herbal formulas that they feel are specific to you that may also improve your sleep.

Massage can also be very helpful. Getting a therapeutic massage on a regular basis can also be very helpful for lowering the threshold of tension to allow you to sleep.

Mind-body therapies. All of the following therapies have been found to be helpful for sleep. The idea that relaxation can actually lead to improved quality of sleep is well founded and supported by the use of these therapies.

- Qi gong
- Tai chi
- Yoga
- Mindfulness meditation
- Cognitive behavioral therapy

16

HERBAL MEDICINE FOR PAIN RELIEF

My interest in writing this chapter is to offer some non-pharmacological approaches for the management of acute and chronic pain. Pain can be a major contributor to mood disorders and can limit activities, relationships, and dramatically interfere with the quality of one's life. Mood disorders also worsen the subjective experience of chronic pain, creating a vicious cycle.

Physical Treatments for Pain Management

Following are non-pharmacological approaches for pain relief.

Osteopathic Manual Therapy and Cranial Osteopathy

I spent the first half of my career dedicating myself to the practice of osteopathic manual medicine and medical acupuncture. These fields of practice are grossly underutilized. It is a true loss in the care of the patient.

Osteopathy is America's best kept medical secret. This is a tragedy since the manual medicine offered by a well-trained osteopathic physician is extraordinary. The manual techniques are varied, applied according to the needs of the patient, and can be incredibly healing. The founder of osteopathy, A.T. Still, understood that the body is a self-healing, self-regulating mechanism, that structure and function are related, and that the body is a whole—all body parts are interactive with each other. The goal of the osteopathic physician is to remove the barriers to healing and allow the body to heal.

I highly recommend anyone with a pain problem to seek out an osteopathic physician who specializes in manual therapy. Cranial osteopathy is a highly specialized, very sophisticated manual therapy with profound effects on the body's ability to heal. Finding a physician trained in both will provide the best treatment.

Here are organizations and websites to find a practitioner in your area:

The American Academy of Osteopathy;
www.americanacademyofosteopathy.org

The Sutherland Cranial Teaching Foundation;
www.sctf.com

The Osteopathic Cranial Academy;
www.cranialacademy.com

Medical Acupuncture and Neuropuncture

Medical acupuncture is taught by Dr. Joseph Helms through the Helms Medical Institute. The type of acupuncture that Dr. Helms teaches is acupuncture energetics, as opposed to traditional Chinese acupuncture. Acupuncture energetics is based on ancient texts brought from China to France to be translated.

This beautiful fusion offers acupuncture in the support of the body's natural healing with acupuncture in the service of modern medicine. Dr. Helms is a fabulous teacher and has a way of elegantly weaving the feeling and the wisdom of ancient Chinese medicine into Western medicine. All of the components of acupuncture are taught: the use of the needles; electroacupuncture; moxa; gua sha (scraping of the skin); auricular and scalp acupuncture; and cupping (the use of cups to increase circulation and cause muscular relaxation).

Medical acupuncture is particularly useful in the treatment of pain, both acute and chronic. Acute pain is easily improved through specific, targeted, meridian-based treatments leading to reduced swelling, pain relief, and rapid healing. But medical acupuncture can also be enormously beneficial for chronic pain. Since pain is experienced in the periphery of the body and sent to the brain through the spinal cord, needles can be strategically placed, and electricity can be strategically applied so the signals from the spinal cord to the brain can be slowed, reducing the experience of the pain. This particular technique is called percutaneous electrical nerve stimulation or PENS and was developed by Dr. Bill Craig. Dr. Helms teaches this technique to physicians through his pain module.

To find a practitioner trained in medical acupuncture go to the American Academy of Medical Acupuncture; www.medicalacupuncture.org.

Michael Corradino, Doctor of Acupuncture and Oriental Medicine, has also discovered the benefits of percutaneous electrical stimulation. He calls his system neuropuncture. The neuropuncture techniques are also designed to use the needles, strategically placed, and electricity strategically applied so the signals from the spinal cord to the brain can be slowed, reducing the experience of the pain. Michael Corradino teaches this particular system to non-physician acupuncturists through Neuropuncture LLC and Healthy Seminars, an online acupuncture training website.

To find a practitioner that Mike has taught in this valuable system, go to www.neuropuncture.com.

Rapid Acupuncture

Rapid acupuncture was developed by Richard Niemtzow, MD, PhD, MPH. By utilizing functional MRI techniques, Dr. Niemtzow was able to identify points on the ear that correlate to organs and body areas. His techniques were developed for the battlefield and are known as battlefield acupuncture. His techniques are not limited to the battlefield and are immensely helpful for migraine headache, dry eyes and mouth, and all types of pain.

This particular type of acupuncture is most commonly offered through the military. If you are a member of the military ask your primary practitioner for a referral.

Myofascial Release

Originally an osteopathic technique, myofascial release is now performed by physicians and physical therapists. This technique consists of maneuvering the body in such a way that the muscles (myo) and their connective tissue (fascia) relax and allow for improved movement of the body and reduced pain. This technique can be very helpful when performed well. It is particularly helpful with excessive muscle tension and in reducing the muscular and fascial strains that follow an accident or injury.

John Barnes, PT, is responsible for promoting and teaching the myofascial release technique and has made it more accessible to patients. He has taught hundreds of practitioners and you can find one trained by him on his website; www.myofascialrelease.com.

Massage

Massage is a time-honored approach for the relief of pain, especially if the pain is located in the muscle. Massage has been practiced by all cultures and around the world and is now available by massage therapists at health spas, salons, in many airports, and even in some shopping malls. The techniques vary depending on who you see, how they are trained and the style that you request. Hot stone massage is a particular favorite of mine, especially when combined with deep massage techniques. There is also shiatsu, reflexology, Swedish massage, and many others.

You can find a good massage therapist most easily by word of mouth. You can start with a local salon and go from there. Ask questions about the different styles of therapy the salon may offer and decide which one fits your needs.

Something that can be done at home that is very helpful for relieving muscle spasm is a castor oil pack. The pack can be placed over the sore area, such as the lower back and worn for an hour. It can be very relieving.

Directions for making a castor oil pack will vary depending on who you ask. I like to make things that are practical, simple, and relatively clean. The biggest difficulty with the pack is that the castor oil is messy and needs to be contained. Here is my preferred method:

Choose a clean white cloth. You want to use a white cloth which has no color or dyes to penetrate into your skin. Flannel is traditionally used, but even a white washcloth or hand towel could work. Fold the cloth in half length-wise so it forms a rectangular shape. Place the cloth on a piece of plastic wrap that is a couple of inches larger than the cloth all around. Fold the plastic edges onto the edge of the cloth, first folding the long edge then the short edge. Tape the plastic to the cloth. This will give the pack a little bit more stability and prevent the oil from soiling anything. Pour the castor oil along the center of the cloth. You will notice that it is thick and does not penetrate into the cloth quickly. Give it some time, maybe 30 minutes, to penetrate and then it is ready for use. Place the pack over the sore area, cloth side down. Place a heating pad or a hot water bottle over the plastic side of the pack. I like to place a thin cloth (like a tee shirt) over the pack to prevent it from sticking to the hot water bottle. Rest with it in place for at least an hour.

For muscle spasm you can add 3–4 drops of essential oil of black pepper into the oil as it saturates the cloth. Black pepper essential oil is extremely relaxing to the muscle. You can also mix in some lobelia oil along with the castor oil pack to help relieve the spasm. The lobelia oil is made by simply pouring oil such as almond oil or grapeseed oil over the lobelia herb and let steep for two weeks. Then the lobelia oil is ready to use. You can also add a small amount of tincture of herbs with muscle relaxing properties. See below for examples. You will find this combination to be most rewarding.

If you are having spasm of the intestines, add some fennel essential oil to the pack. Fennel essential oil is an excellent relaxant of smooth muscle. Use 3–4 drops per pack and mix into the castor oil, allowing it to penetrate. Place the castor oil pack over the belly and rest with the heat source covering the pack.

Herbals for Pain Management

Due to the opiate epidemic, opiate treatment for chronic pain is not the best choice. Acupuncture has been incredibly helpful in relieving pain without the use of opiates and also helps people come off opiate medication. Herbal medicine can also be useful. What follows is a list of herbal remedies that are helpful for pain, organized by pain location and type.

Herbs to Use for Pain That Interferes with Sleep

California poppy (*Eschscholzia californica*). This is always the first herb that comes to my mind when someone cannot sleep because of pain. California poppy binds to both opiate receptors and to GABA receptors so it causes both relaxation and pain relief. California poppy is one of many herbals used in the management of opiate withdrawal. It will give you a positive opiate urine test, so keep that in mind if you are drug tested in the workplace. Follow the directions on the product that you purchase. Secrets of the Tribe and Hawaii Pharm both have alcohol free tinctures. Since California poppy is sedating and relaxing it is used during the day in small doses and a larger dose before bed.

Turkey corn (*Corydalis cava, C spp.*). This herb is commonly used for pain. There are many species in the corydalis family, and all have value. Corydalis cava is also known by its Chinese name *Yanhusuo* also seen as *Yan hu suo*. The corydalis species have action on the opiate receptors and has been shown to be effective specifically for nerve pain. Purchase online and follow the directions on the product that you purchase.

Jamaican dogwood (*Piscidia piscipula, P. erythrina*). Jamaican dogwood has mild narcotic effects and it is sedating, so it is useful for pain-disrupted sleep. It is toxic if used long term so limit daily use to fourteen days. It has an affinity for nerve pain in the trigeminal nerve, a very severe pain for those who have the affliction. It also has an affinity for pain in the nerves of the neck. It is useful for the pain of migraine headaches, insomnia due to nervous tension, and stress. For dosing, follow the directions on the bottle of the product that you purchase. It combines well with corydalis; a mixture of 4-parts corydalis and 1-part Jamaican dogwood can be very helpful for getting you through an exacerbation of a pain complaint. Jamaican dogwood cannot be used for more than two weeks in a row due to possible toxicity.

Anti-Inflammatory Herbs

There are many herbs that have anti-inflammatory effects. This is a partial list of anti-inflammatory herbs with a general action or a specific focus on musculoskeletal inflammation that deserve special mention.

White peony (*Paeonia lactiflora*). This is a remarkably effective anti-inflammatory herb. For those who are familiar with the beautiful and aromatic white peony blossoms, please understand that the tincture is made from the root of the plant, not the flower. The tincture is called white when the bark is removed from the root. It has been used in Asian countries for

1200 years to treat muscle spasm, fever, and autoimmune diseases of the joints and connective tissues such as rheumatoid
arthritis and systemic lupus erythematosus. I find the relief from
the tincture or glycerite is almost immediate and the immobil-
ity of an arthritic joint resolves quickly. White peony also has
some anti-spasmodic effects.

I have osteoarthritis fairly severely and have had it since I
was young. While writing this book, at the end of a day of typ-
ing all day, my right shoulder would be so painful that I would
be unable to use my arm. I would literally have to use my left
hand to lift my right hand to the keyboard. One particular day
like that, I was not able to move my arm and the pain was a 10
on a scale of pain 1–10. I took a dropperful of white peony and a
dropperful of corydalis and within minutes I could feel the pain
receding and I had full use of my arm. Not everyone has that
same response, but I find it to be a fairly reliable herbal remedy
for acute pain. Follow the directions on the bottle of the product
you purchase.

Frankincense (*Boswellia serrate*). Used since ancient
times for the management of pain, frankincense has anti-
inflammatory actions on the joints and surrounding tissues
such as ligaments and tendons, as well as on the gastrointestinal tract. It is available as a standardized extract capsule of
50 percent to 60 percent boswellic acids. Take 1000 mg three
times daily. To reach the effective dose consider a powder form:
dosage of most formulas is too low.

Turmeric (*Turmeric longa*). Used for centuries as an
anti-inflammatory, turmeric is an effective anti-inflammatory
for the gut when consumed alone. If the desired effect is to
reduce inflammation in the rest of the body, it must be consumed

with fat and pepper or a pepper extract, commonly sold as bio-perine. Be sure to purchase the type of product for the desired action. Follow the directions on the bottle of the product that you purchase.

Ginger (*Zingiber officinale*). Ginger is well known as an anti-inflammatory herb. It is common for turmeric, Boswellia, and ginger to be mixed in an over-the-counter supplement. The combination of these three herbals can be very effective. Follow the directions on the bottle of the product that you choose.

For Neuropathy

Dr. Jill Stansbury, in her book *Psychiatry and Pain Management*, recommends the following herbal remedy:

> *Curcuma longa* (turmeric)
>
> *Zingiber officinalis* (ginger)
>
> *Corydalis yanhusuo* or *C. cava* (corydalis)
>
> *Harpagophytum procumbens* (devil's claw)
>
> *Gingko biloba* (gingko)

Mix equal parts of tincture or alcohol-free tincture into a bottle. Take a dropperful (20–30 drops) as needed. Take every hour for acute pain, if needed.

You can purchase all these tinctures online. My go-to for alcohol free is Hawaii Pharm or Secrets of the Tribe.

Low Back Pain and Muscle Spasm

Lobelia (*Lobelia inflate*). Extremely helpful for low back pain, lobelia is especially useful for the muscle spasm that grabs you and won't let you go. The lobelia herb can be infused into oil such as almond oil or safflower oil and applied topically. To infuse oil with an herb, simply pour the oil over the herb and let it sit for two weeks. Strain and use. Lobelia oil is especially useful when used in combination with castor oil for the castor oil pack. You can simply pour the lobelia-infused oil on the castor oil and let them soak into the cloth together. Use as you would any castor oil pack.

If you need a more potent application, vinegar can pull more of the muscle-relaxing constituents out of the dried lobelia leaves. Soak the dried leaves in apple cider vinegar for 15 minutes. Add 2 cups of boiling water over the lobelia and let sit for another 10 minutes. Strain and when cooled, add the lobelia vinegar to the castor oil to make your castor oil pack. Use as you would use any castor oil pack.

There are many herbs that are helpful for reducing muscle spasm. The following are worth special mention.

Cramp bark (*Viburnum opulus*); black haw (*Viburnum prunifolium*). These herbs are best known for their affinity for menstrual cramps; however, they can be helpful for any muscle cramp or spasm. In *A Modern Herbal,* by Mrs. Grieve, these herbs are "used with benefit in cramps and spasms of all kinds, in convulsions, fits, and lock jaw . . ." Cramp bark and black haw are also known as guelder rose and used as a tea, a decoction (simmered herb to make tea), and an extract, and are also available as a supplement. As a tea, cramp bark is slightly bitter but tolerable.

Recently, I was packing to move and did a lot of bending, twisting, and lifting of heavy items for many hours. I predicted I would be sore and stiff the following day so as a precautionary measure, I made a cup of cramp bark tea and consumed a tea-spoonful every 30–60 minutes. I am happy to report it was successful and I had no muscle cramping that evening or the following day.

Black cohosh (*Acteae racemosa*). Best known as the meno-pause herb, it has been used historically for rheumatic pain, muscle spasm, and tension. It is commercially available as the herb (which makes a bitter tea), as an extract, and as a supple-ment. The supplement is advertised for menopause, but it will work for your pain as well. Follow the directions on the product that you purchase.

Lobelia inflate. See above.

All the herbs listed for tension headache below would also be helpful for muscle spasm.

Essential Oil Cream for Topical Pain Relief

Use a suitable oil carrier such as coconut oil. Place in a 6-ounce glass container. Add 3 drops of the following essential oils: Black pepper, Lavender, Roman chamomile, and Rosemary, and 2 drops of Cinnamon and Peppermint. Combine well and apply liberally to affected area as often as needed. You can vary the essential oils and their doses according to your preferences.

Tension Headache

Wood betony (*Stachys officinalis*). Excellent for tension headaches, it is best taken as a tincture or a tea. The tea has a pleasant vanilla aftertaste and I recommend adding a drop of vanilla extract to boost the flavor. Start with 3–4 cups daily for 2 weeks and as the headache subsides reduce the dose of the tea to 1 to 2 cups daily. This herb is also excellent for the headache following head injury.

Tension Headache Tincture by Dr. Jill Stansbury

Dr. Stansbury has a recipe for tension headache tea that is quite effective. You can make the tincture by purchasing the individual tinctures and mixing them together as indicated in the recipe or you can ask a community herbalist to make the tinctures for you. Be mindful that tinctures are most commonly made with alcohol. There are alcohol free alternatives available if you want to avoid using an alcohol-based product. My go-to for alcohol free products is Hawaii Pharm or Secrets of the Tribe.

Tincture for muscle tension headaches

Mix together the following tinctures (1 teaspoon equals 5 ml):

10 ml kava (*Piper methysticum*)

10 ml California poppy (*Eschscholzia californica*)

10 ml black cohosh (*Actaea racemosa*)

10 ml *Corydalis cava*

10 ml Jamaican dogwood (*Piscidia piscipula*)

10 ml *Rauwolfia serpentine*

Take 1 teaspoon of the mixture three times a day. Take 1 teaspoon every 15 minutes for acute muscle spasms and tension headache. Reduce the dose as symptoms improve.

(Dr. Jill Stansbury, *Herbal Formularies for Health Professionals, Volume 4, Neurology, Psychiatry and Pain Management*, p. 164.)

A note about Rauwolfia: This product is not available as a typical tincture. It is only sold as a homeopathic mother tincture. The mother tincture is the original botanical tincture from which other homeopathics are made. It is made with 65 percent grain alcohol. *Do not* consume it on its own; always mix it with other products.

Migraine Headache

Magnesium. Migraine headache and magnesium go hand in hand; 400–600 mg of magnesium picolinate daily is helpful. These higher doses may cause loose stools and if that happens reduce the dose.

Butterbur (*Petisites hybridus*). 75 mg daily is helpful for migraine headache prevention. *Petisites* contains a compound nicknamed PA (pyrolyzing alkaloids), which are considered toxic, especially to young children. Purchase products that are PA free.

Feverfew (*Tenacetum parthenium*).Butterbur is often combined with feverfew. The early research on feverfew showed that it was most effective if it was consumed fresh, either as a tea or a tincture made from the fresh plant. However, most products sold in the marketplace are of the dried variety. The research on the dried plant is less compelling although I have a few patients who find the feverfew very helpful.

Arthritic Joint Pain

Ginger poultice is helpful for the painful joint and can also improve joint function. A poultice is made using a cloth similar to one used in the castor oil pack. To the cloth add grated, frozen, fresh ginger root. When it is grated it will put off a liquid and the ginger will be able to be spread onto the cloth. The cloth can then be placed on the sore joint and wrapped to keep it in place. This may be worn overnight. When there is inflammation, the poultice will get hot and you should keep it on as long as it is tolerable. The ginger poultice will relieve the pain, the swelling, and improve joint function.

All the herbs that are anti-inflammatory or pain relieving can be used for arthritic pain. Black cohosh that is mentioned above is very helpful for arthritic pain in both osteoarthritis and in the rheumatoid arthritis types.

Supplements Commonly Used for the Treatment of Osteoarthritis

Glucosamine, chondroitin, and MSM are commonly sold together as supplements. This is what the research shows:

Chondroitin sulfate demonstrates improvement in disease progression, pain, and measurable joint function. As stated, it is commonly sold in combination with glucosamine and MSM, but it is sold on its own by Source Naturals. Take 600 mg, three times daily.

Glucosamine improves stiffness but not disease progression. Available in combination products.

MSM (methylsulfonylmethane) is better than placebo for pain and function but not stiffness. However, the dose used in the study is 6 grams daily; 3 grams twice a day. Most products sold over the counter use much smaller doses. If using MSM, consider the powder and adjust the dose to be equivalent to 3 grams twice daily.

Pau d'arco (*Tabebuia avellanedae*). Pau d'arco tincture was found to be protective of the cartilage and underlying bone and provided pain relief and improved function. Available in tincture and alcohol-free tinctures online. Follow the directions on the bottle of the product that you purchase.

FINAL THOUGHTS

Herbal medicine is a time-honored medicine which is still widely used around the world today. We can say that it is traditional medicine having been used by various cultures around the world and long before pharmaceutical medications became available.

Herbal medicine offers remedies that are more gentle, effective, and have fewer side effects than the more powerful and harsh pharmaceuticals.

I love herbal medicine, and herbs are used widely in my own home for everything from a bug bite to a sleeping aide. It is amazing to me that we can grow a sedative such as valerian (*Valeriana*), harvest it and consume it, and get relief from anxiety. Or grow skullcap (*Scutellaria lateriflora*) in the yard and make it into a relaxing tea that is delicious and soothing. Mullein grows wild in my neighborhood, and when I need a cough remedy I can just go out and pick it.

Herbs have their own indications and personalities. It takes study and experience to utilize them effectively. When a pharmaceutical medication is needed, it should be used appropriately. But the wide world of herbal medicine offers a great many alternatives and opportunities for safe and effective care, right from the garden.

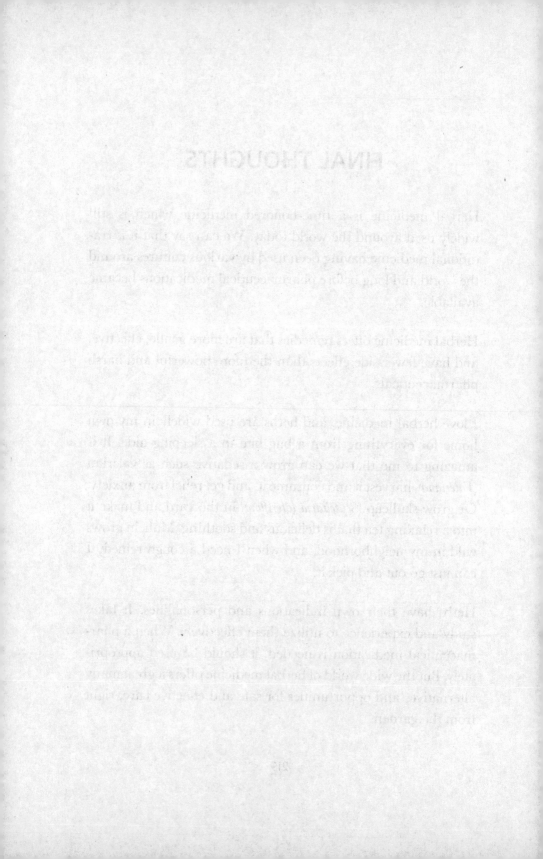

ENDNOTES

1. *"Chef's Guide" to Herbs and Spices*, Jay Weinstein, BarCharts Publishing, Inc. © 2018.

2. Thomas Easley, *The Modern Herbal Dispensatory*, Steven Horne North Atlantic Books, 297.

3. James Duke, PhD, *Handbook of Medicinal Herbs*, 2002 CRC Press, 640.

4. www.ncbi.nlm.nih.gov/pubmed/?term=bacopa+monnieri+thyroid.

5. thyroidadvisor.com/bacopa-monnieri-effects-benefits-thyroid-gland.

6. pubmed.ncbi.nlm.nih.gov/11783267.

7. Ginseng on hypothyroidism in rats: pubmed.ncbi.nlm.nih.gov/29021704/?from_term=red+ginseng+and+thyroid&from_pos=1.

8. Dr. Sharol Marie Tilgner, "Herbal Medicine from The Heart of the Earth," 3rd edition, edited by Louis Fiore, Wise Acres, LLC, 2020, 52.

9. www.nih.gov/news-events/news-releases/panel-recommends-changing-name-common-disorder-women.

10. www.ncbi.nlm.nih.gov/pubmed/18950759.

11. www.ncbi.nlm.nih.gov/pmc/articles/PMC4963579.

12. Ibid.

13. Vitamin D in Dementia and MCI: www.ncbi.nlm.nih.gov/pubmed/32248358; Vitamin D and Cognition and maintaining muscle strength: Muir S.W., et al., *Journal of the American Geriatric Society* 2011, 59(12): 2291–3000; Vitamin D and Colon cancer survival; lower mortality every 10 ng/ml your D goes up it confers 29 percent improvement of mortality: Weinstein S.J., et al., *International Journal of Cancer* 2014; doi:10.1002/ijc.29157; Muscle strength and longevity, articles.mercola.com/sites/articles/archive/2020/03/14/

skeletal-muscle-aging.aspx; Vitamin D Improves Breast Cancer Survival: Kim Y, et al., *British Journal of Cancer* 2014, 110(11): 2772–2784; Jacobs E.T., et al., *Journal of Cancer* 2016, 7(3): 232–240; Vitamin D is an anti-zinflammatory and improves endothelial function with reduction of MI risk: Giovannucci E,, et al., *Archives of Internal Medicine* 2008, 168: 1174–1180; Cavalho L.S., et al., *Atherosclerosis* 2015, 241(2): 729.

14. Dale Bredesen, *The End of Alzheimer's.* Penguin Publishing Group, Kindle Edition, 121–123.

15. www.sepalika.com/type-2-diabetes/gymnema-sylvestre-diabetes.

16. M. Fennell, Cognitive behaviour therapy for depressive disorders. In M. Gelder, N. Andreasen, J. Lopez-Ibor, and J. Geddes, editors, *New Oxford Textbook of Psychiatry*. New York: Oxford University Press, 2012, 1304–1312. [Google Scholar]

17. www.ncbi.nlm.nih.gov/pmc/articles/PMC2933381.

18. www.ncbi.nlm.nih.gov/pmc/articles/PMC7144187.

19. www.alpha-stim.com/healthcare-professionals/research-and-reports-2-2/

20. The research bibliography can be found here: www.interactivemetronome.com/images/pdfs/IM-RESEARCH-BIBLIOGRAPHY.pdf.

21. connect.hyperbaricmedicalsolutions.com/hubfs/HyperbaricMedicalSolutions_July2018/Docs/A-Phase-I-Study-of-Low-Pressure-Hyperbaric-Oxygen-Therapy-for-Blast-Induced-Post-Concussion-Syndrome-and-Post-Traumatic-Stress-Disorder.pdf.

22. www.ncbi.nlm.nih.gov/pmc/articles/PMC4610617.

23. jissn.biomedcentral.com/articles/10.1186/1550-2783-10-37.

24. Christopher Hobbs, *Stress and Natural Healing*, Interweave Press, 207.

25. David Winston, RH (AHG) and Steven Maimes, *Adaptogens, Herbs for Strength, Stamina and Stress Relief*, Rochester, Vermont: Healing Arts Press, 2007 and 2019, 157–161.

26. Stephen P. Hinshaw, *Annual Review of Clinical Psychology* 2018. 14: 291–316.

27. Dvořáková M., Ježová D., Blažíček P., et al. *Nutrition Neuroscience* 2007, 10(3–4): 151–157; doi: 10.1080/09513590701565443.

28. Zuzana Chovanová 1, Jana Muchová, Monika Sivonová, Monika Dvoráková, Ingrid Zitnanová, Iveta Waczulíková, Jana Trebatická, Igor Skodácek, Zdenka Duracková, *Free Radical Research* 2006, Sep. 40(9): 1003–1010; doi: 10.1080/10715760600824902.

29. BlueCross BlueShield, The Impact of Attention Deficit Disorder on the Health of American Children. (2019 March 28).

30. R. Bluth, ADHD numbers are rising and scientists are trying to understand why, *Washington Post.* (2018 Sept 10).

31. *Annual Review of Clinical Psychology* 2018, 14: 291–316.

32. *Annual Review of Clinical Psychology* 2018, 14: 293.

33. pubmed.ncbi.nlm.nih.gov/29165401/?from_term=bacopa+monnieri+and+attention&from_pos=3.

34. pubmed.ncbi.nlm.nih.gov/27912958/?from_term=bacopa+monnieri+and+attention&from_pos=4.

35. pubmed.ncbi.nlm.nih.gov/23195757.

36. Bradwejn, J., Zhou, Y., Koszycki, D., and Shlik, J. A double-blind, placebo-controlled study on the effects of Gotu kola (*Centella asiatica*) on acoustic startle response in healthy subjects. *Journal of Clinical Psychopharmacology* 2000, 20: 680–684.

37. www.banyanbotanicals.com/info/plants/ayurvedic-herbs/mucuna-pruriens.

38. Dvořáková, M., Ježová, D., Blažíček, P., et al. *Nutrition Neuroscience* 2007, 10(3–4):151–157; doi: 10.1080/09513590701565443.

39. Chovanová, Z., Muchová, J., Sivonová, M., Dvoráková, M., Zitnanová, I., Waczulíková, I., et al., *Free Radical Research* 2006, Sep. 40(9): 1003–1010; doi: 10.1080/10715760600824902.z

REFERENCES

Agusti A, Garcia-Pardo M P, López-Almela I, Campillo I, Maes M, Romani-Pérez M, Sanz Y: Interplay between the gut-brain axis, obesity and cognitive function. *Front Neuroscience* (2018) 12: 155 www.ncbi.nlm.nih.gov/pmc/articles/PMC5864897.

Alpha-stim.com: www.alpha-stim.com/healthcare-professionals/research-and-reports-2-2.

Amen, Daniel MD: Healing ADD: *The Breakthrough Program that Allows You to See and Heal the 7 Types of ADD*. New York: The Berkley Publishing Group, Penguin Random House, 2015.

Amen, Daniel MD and Routh, Lisa C MD: *Healing Anxiety and Depression*. New York: The Berkley Publishing Group, Penguin Random House, 2003.

American Botanical Council: Proprietary Botanical Ingredient Scientific and Clinical Monograph for Pycogenol (French Maritime Pine Bark Extract) *Pinus pinaster* Aiton Subsp. *Atlantica* [FamPinacea] 2019 Update. abc.herbalgram.org/site/DocServer/Pycnog_FullMono012019-final-FULL.pdf;jsessionid=00000000.app20051b?docID=8983&NONCE_TOKEN=A316C1A89C5C9C5B97DDD77FE18A7BA1.

Baek J H, Nierenberg A, Kinrys G: Clinical applications for herbal medicines for anxiety and insomnia; targeting patients with bipolar disorder. *Australia New Zealand Journal of Psychiatry* (Aug. 2014) 48(8): 705–715. doi: 10.1177/0004867414539198.Epub 2014 Jun 19. pubmed.ncbi.nlm.nih.gov/24947278.

Bair M J, Robinson R L, Katon W, Kroenke K: Depression and pain comorbidity: A literature review. *Archives of Internal Medicine* (Nov. 10, 2003) 163(20): 2433–2445. doi: 10.1001/archinte.163.20.2433; pubmed.ncbi.nlm.nih.gov/14609780.

Bandelow B: Epidemiology of anxiety disorders in the 21st century. *Diaglogues Clinical Neuroscience* (Sept. 17, 2015) (3): 327–335.www.ncbi.nlm.nih.gov/pmc/articles/PMC4610617/

Banyanbotanicals.com: The Benefits of Macuna Puriens, updated 2020. www.banyanbotanicals.com/info/plants/ayurvedic-herbs/mucuna-pruriens.

Bartholomew J, Linder D: State anxiety following resistance exercise: The role of gender and exercise intensity. *Journal of Behavioral Medicine* (Apr. 21, 1998) 205–219. link.springer.com/article/10.1023/A:1018732025340.

Benelli E, Del Ghianda S, Di Cosmo C, Tonacchera M: A combined therapy with myo-inositol and D-chiro-inositol improves endocrine parameters and insulin resistance in PCOS young overweight women. *International Journal of Endocrinology* (2016) 3204083. www.ncbi.nlm.nih.gov/pmc/articles/PMC4963579.

Benzie IFF, Wachtel-Galor S, editors: *Herbal Medicine: Biomolecular and Clinical Aspects.* 2nd edition. Boca Raton, FL: CRC Press, 2011. Bookshelf ID: NBK92750PMID: 22593920.

Berg B, Roos E M, Englund M, Kise N J, Tiulpin A, Saarakkala S, Engebretsen L, Eftang C N, Holm I, Risberg M A: Development of osteoarthritis in patients with degenerative meniscal tears treated with exercise therapy or surgery: A Randomized Controlled Trial. *Osteoarthritis Cartilage* (Mar. 2006) 14(3): 286–294. doi: 10.1016/j.joca.2005.10.003. Epub 2005 Nov 23. pubmed.ncbi.nlm.nih.gov/32184135.

Bhattacharya S K, Ghosal S: Anxiolytic activity of a standardized extract of *Bacopa monnieri*: An experimental study. *Phytomedicine* (Apr. 1998) 5(2): 77–82. doi: 10.1016/S0944-7113(98)80001-9 pubmed.ncbi.nlm.nih.gov/23195757.

BioNET-EAFRINET Keys and Fact Sheets: Avena fatua (Common Wild Oat) keys.lucidcentral.org/keys/v3/eafrinet/weeds/key/weeds/Media/Html/Avena_fatua_(Common_Wild_Oat).htm.

Bjørklund G, Hilt B, Dadar M, Lindh U, Aaseth J: Neurotoxic effects of mercury exposure in dental personnel. *Review Basic Clinical Pharmacological Toxicology* (May 2019) 124(5): 568–574. Doi 10.111/bcpt.13199. PMID: 30589214. doi: 10.1111/bcpt.13199.

Bone, Kerry ND: *Clinical Applications of Ayurvedic and Chinese Herbs, Monographs for the Western Herbal Practitioner.* Third printing. Warwick, Queensland, 4370, Australia: Phytotherapy Press, 2000.

Bradwejn J, Zhou Y, Koszycki D, Shlik J: A double-blind, placebo-controlled study on the effects of Gotu kola (*Centella Asiatica*) on acoustic startle response in healthy subjects. *Journal of Clinical Psychopharmacology* (2000) 20:680–684.

Bredesen, DE MD: *The End of Alzheimer's, The First Program to Prevent and Reverse Cognitive Decline.* New York: Avery, an imprint of Penguin Random House, 2017.

Brown, Richard MD and Gerbarg, Patricia L MD: *Non-Drug Treatments for ADHD.* New York: W.W. Norton and Company, 2012.

Bystritsky A, Kerwin L, Feusner J D: A pilot study of *Rhodiola rosea* (Rhodax) for generalized anxiety disorder (GAD). *Journal of Alternative Complementary Medicine* (Mar. 2008) 14(2): 175–180. doi: 10.1089/acm.2007.7117 www.ncbi.nlm.nih.giv/pubmed/18307390.

Calabrese C, Gregory W, Leo M, Kraemer D, Bone K, Oken B: Effects of a standardized *Bacopa monnieri* extract on cognitive performance, anxiety, and depression in the elderly: A randomized, double-blind, placebo-controlled trial. *Journal of Alternative Complementary Medicine* (Jul. 2008) 14(6): 707–713. www.ncbi.nlm.nih.gov/pmc/articles/PMC3153866.

Camfield D A, Stough C, Farrimond J, Scholey A B: Acute effect to tea constituents l-theanine, caffeine, and epigallocatechin gallate on cognitive function and mood: A systematic review and meta-analysis. *Nutrition Review* (Aug. 2014) 72(8): 507–522. doi: 10.1111/nure.12120. Epub 2014 Jun 19. pubmed.ncbi.nlm.nih.gov/24946991.

Canadian Research Knowledge Network: Benefits of saffron PDF 16 September 2010. Access details: [subscription number 918588849]. Publisher Taylor & Francis Informa Ltd Registered in England and Wales Registered Number: 1072954 Registered office: Mortimer House, 37-41 Mortimer Street, London W1T 3JH, UK.

Catrin L, Roberts N P, Andrew M, Starling E, Bisson J: Psychological therapies for post-traumatic stress disorder in adults: A systematic review and meta-analysis. *European Journal of Psychotraumatology* (2020) 11(1): 1729633. www.ncbi.nlm.nih.gov/pmc/articles/PMC7144187.

Cavalho LS, et al.: Vitamin d is an anti-inflammatory and improves endothelial function with reduction of MI risk. *Atherosclerosis* (2015) 241(2): 729–740.

Cenit M C, Neuvo, I C, Codoñer-Franch P, Dinan T G, Sanz Y: A key role of the microbiota in neurodevelopmental disorders. Gut microbiota and attention deficit hyperactivity disorder: New perspectives for a challenging condition. *European Child and Adolescent Psychiatry* (2017) 26: 1081–1092.

Chovanová Z, Muchová J, Sivonová M, Dvoráková M, Zitnanová I, Waczulíková I, Trebatická J, Skodácek I, Duracková Z: Effect of ADHD by oxidative stress, reduction of ROS, improved DNA damage of the brain in ADHD children. Effect of polyphenolic extract, pycnogenol, on the level of 8-oxoguanine in children suffering from attention deficit/hyperactivity disorder. *Free Radic Resolution* (Sept. 2006) 40(9): 1003–1010. Doi 10.1080/10715760600824902. pubmed.ncbi.nlm.nih.gov/17015282.

Chutkan, R: *The Microbiome Solution, A Radical New Way to Heal Your Body from the Inside Out.* New York: Penguin Random House, 2015.

Clement K, Covertson C, Johnson MJ, Dearing K: St. John's wort and the treatment of mild to moderate depression: A systematic review. *Holistic Nurse Practitioner* (Jul–Aug 2006) 20(4): 197–203. doi: 10.1097/00004650-200607000-00008. www.ncbi.nlm.nih.gov/pubmed/?term=16825922.

Dai X, Zhou Y, Yu X: [Effect of ginseng injection in treating congestive heart failure and its influence on thyroid hormones]. *Zhongguo Zhong Xi Yi Jie He Za Zhi* (Apr. 1999) 19(4): 209–211. pubmed.ncbi.nlm.nih.gov/11783267. [Article in Chinese]

DeRubeis R J, Siegle G J, Hollon S D: Cognitive therapy vs. medications for depression: Treatment outcomes and neural mechanisms. *Natural Review Neuroscience* (Oct. 2008) 9(10): 788–796. www.ncbi.nlm.nih.gov/pmc/articles/PMC2748674.

Dietz C, Dekker M: Effect of green tea phytochemicals on mood and cognition. *Current Pharmaceutical Design* (2017) 23(19): 2876–2905. doi: 10.21 74/1381612823666170105151800. pubmed.ncbi.nlm.nih.gov/28056735.

Driessen E, Hollon S: Cognitive behavioral therapy for mood disorders: Efficacy, moderators and mediators. *Psychiatric Clinics of North America* (Sept. 2010) 33(3): 537–555. www.ncbi.nlm.nih.gov/pmc/articles/PMC2933381.

Drugs.com: Saffron.www.drugs.com/npp/saffron.html.

Dvořáková M, Ježová D, Blažíček P, et al.: Urinary catecholamines in children with attention deficit hyperactivity disorder (ADHD): Modulation by a polyphenolic extract from pine bark (Pycnogenol). *Nutrition Neuroscience* (2007) 10(3–4): 151–157. doi: 10.1080/09513590701565443. pubmed. ncbi.nlm.nih.gov/16984739.

Dvoráková M, Sivonová M, Trebatická J, Skodácek I, Waczuliková I, Muchová J, Ducková Z: The effect of polyphenolic pine bark, Pycnogenol on the level of glutathione in children suffering from attention deficit hyperactivity disorder (ADHD). *Redox Report* (2006) 11(4): 163–172. doi: 10.1179/135100006X116664 pubmed.ncbi.nlm.nih.gov/16984739.

Easley, Thomas and Horne, Steven: *The Modern Herbal Dispensatory, A Medicine Making Guide*. Berkeley, CA: North Atlantic Books, 2016.

Edelman, Eva: *Natural Healing for Schizophrenia and Other Common Mental Disorders*. Eugene, OR: Borage Books, 1996, 1998, 2001.

Edison T: Thomas Edison's seminal invention of the electric light bulb in 1879 brought unprecedented possibilities, and the American inventor is attributed with once remarking, "The doctor of the future will give no medicine, but will instruct his patient in the care of the human frame, in diet, and in the cause and prevention of disease."

Ekor M: Nephrotoxicity and nephroprotective potential of African medicinal plants. *Toxicological Survey of African Medicinal Plants* (2014). www. sciencedirect.com/topics/agricultural-and-biological-sciences/dioscorea.

Endocrine Society: Treating vitamin D deficiency may improve depression. *ScienceDaily*. (June 25, 2012). www.sciencedaily.com/ releases/2012/06/120625152358.htm.

Eymundsdottir H, Chang M, Geirsdottir O G, Gudmundsson L S, Jonsson P V, Gudnason V, Launer, Jonssorrier M K, Ramel A: Lifestyle and 25-hydroxy-vitamin D among community-dwelling old adults with dementia, mild cognitive impairment, or normal cognitive function. *Aging Clinical and Experimental Research* (Dec. 2020) 32(12): 2649–2656. doi: 10.1007/s40520-020-01531-1.Epub 2020 Apr 4. www.ncbi.nlm.nih.gov/ pubmed/32248358.

Farrell, D: *Herbs for Depression and Anxiety, Learn How to Relieve the Symptoms of Depression and Anxiety, Anxiety Disorder, Panic Attacks and Stress Management*. Self Published, 2016.

Fennell M: "Cognitive Behaviour Therapy for Depressive Disorders. New Oxford Textbook of Psychiatry." Gelder M, Andreasen N, Lopez-Ibor J,

Geddes J, editors. New York: Oxford University Press, 2012, pp. 1304–1312. [Google Scholar]

Gautam M, Tripathi A, Deshmukh D, Gaur M: Cognitive behavior therapy for depression. *Indian Journal of Psychiatry* (Jan. 2020) 62(Suppl 2): S223–S229. www.ncbi.nlm.nih.gov/pmc/articles/PMC7001356/#ref2.

Gershon, M D, M.D.: *The Second Brain, Your Gut Has a Mind of Its Own, A Groundbreaking New Understanding of Nervous Disorders of the Stomach and Intestine.* New York, London, Toronto, Sydney: Harper, 1998.

Giovannucci E, Liu Y, Hollis B, Rimm R: 25-hydroxyvitamin D and risk of myocardial infarction in men: A prospective study. *Archives of Internal Medicine* (2008) 168: 1174–1180.

Gourbeye P, Berri M, Lippi Y, Meurens F, Vincent-Naulleau S, Laffitte J, Rogel-Gaillard C, Pinton P, Oswald I: Pattern recognition receptors in the gut: analysis of their expression along the intestinal tract and the crypt/villus axis. *Physiology Report* (Feb. 2015) 3(2): e12225. www.ncbi.nlm.nih.gov/pmc/articles/PMC4393184.

Gray S, Meijer R, Barrett E: Insulin regulates brain function but how does it get there? *Diabetes* (Dec. 2014) 63(12): 3992–3997. doi.org/10.2337/db14-0340. diabetes.diabetesjournals.org/content/63/12/3992.

Grieve, M: *A Modern Herbal, The Medicinal, Culinary, Cosmetic and Economic Properties, Cultivation and Folk-Lore of Herbs, Grasses, Fungi, Shrubs and Trees with All their Modern Scientific Uses.* In two volumes. Garden City, NY: Dover Publications, 1971.

Guan S-Y, Zhang K, Wang X-S, Yang L, Feng B, Tain D-D, Gao M-R, Liu S-B, Liu A, Zhao M-G: Anxiolytic effects of polydatin through the blockade of neuroinflammation in a chronic pain mouse model. *Molecular Pain* (Jan–Dec 2020) 16:1744806919900717. doi: 10.1177/1744806919900717 pubmed.ncbi.nlm.nih.gov/31964240.

Guyol, Gracelyn: *Healing Depression and Bipolar Disorder Without Drugs.* New York: Walker and Company, 2006.

Harch, P G, et al.: A Phase I study of low-pressure hyperbaric oxygen therapy for blast-induced post-concussion syndrome and post-traumatic stress disorder. *Journal of Neurotrauma* (Jan. 12, 2012) 29: 168–185, Mary Ann Liebert, Inc. doi: 10.1089/neu.2011.1895. connect.hyperbaricmedicalsolutions.com/hubfs/HyperbaricMedicalSolutions_July2018/Docs/A-Phase-I-Study-of-Low-Pressure-Hyperbaric-Oxygen-Therapy-for-Blast-Induced-Post-Concussion-Syndrome-and-Post-Traumatic-Stress-Disorder.pdf.

Hartvigsen J, et al.: What low back pain is and why we need to pay attention. *Lancet* (Jun 9, 2018) 391(10137): 2356–2367. doi: 10.1016/S0140-6736(18)30480-X.Epub 2018 Mar 21. pubmed.ncbi.nlm.nih.gov/29573870.

Hedaya R J: *The Antidepressant Survival Guide.* New York: Three Rivers Press, Member of the Crown Publishing Group, 2000.

Hinshaw S P: Attention deficit hyperactivity disorder (ADHD): Controversy, developmental mechanisms, and multiple levels of analysis. *Annual Review of Clinical Psychology* (2018) 14: 291–316.

Hobbs, Christopher: *Stress and Natural Healing, Herbal Medicines and Natural Therapies for: Depression, Anxiety, Insomnia, Heart Disease, Herbal support for Prozac, Zoloft and More.* Loveland, CO: Botanica Press, an imprint for Interweave Press, Inc., 1997.

Holmes, Peter: *The Energetics of Western Herbs, A Materia Medica Integrating Western and Chinese Herbal Therapeutics.* Vol. 1 and Vol. 2, Revised and Enlarged 4th Edition. Cotati, CA: Snow Lotus Press, 1989, 1993, 1997, 2000, 2007.

Huang H-Y, Liao H-Y, Lin Y-W: Effects and mechanisms of electroacupuncture on chronic inflammatory pain and depression comorbidity in mice. *Evid Based Complement Alternative Medicine* (May 2020) 28: 4951591. doi: 10.1155/2020/4951591.eCollection 2020. pubmed.ncbi.nlm.nih.gov/32565863.

Humble M, Gustafsson S, Bejerot S: Low serum levels of 25-hydroxyvitamin D (25-OHD) among psychiatric out-patients in Sweden: Relations with season, age, ethnic origin and psychiatric diagnosis. *Journal of Steroid Biochemistry and Molecular Biology* (Jul. 2010) 121(1–2): 467–470. doi: 10.1016/j.jsbmb.2010.03.013.Epub 2010 Mar 7. www.ncbi.nlm.nih.gov/pubmed/20214992.

Irwin M R: Why sleep is important for health: A psychoneuroimmunology perspective. *Annual Review of Psychology* (Jan. 2015) (3)66: 143–172. doi:10.1146/annurev-psych-010213-115205. www.ncbi.nlm.nih.gov/pmc/articles/PMC4961463/pdf/nihms804179.

Jones E G: *Definite Medication, Containing Therapeutic Facts Gleaned from Forty Years Practice.* Boston, MA: The Therapeutic Publishing Company, 1911.

Kamhi E PHD, RN, HNC and Zampieron E R ND, MH (AHG): *Arthritis, Reverse Underlying Causes of Arthritis with Clinically Proven Alternative Therapies.* New York: Celestial Arts, an imprint of the Crown Publishing Group, a division of Random House, 2006.

Katz M, Levie A, Kol-Degani H, Kav-Venaki L: A compound herbal preparation (CHP) in the treatment of children with ADHD: A randomized controlled trial. *Journal of Attention Disorders* (2010) 14(3): 281–291.

Kean J D, Downey L A, Stough C: Systematic overview of Bacopa monnieri (L.) Wettst. Dominant poly-herbal formulas in children and adolescents. *Medicines (Basel)* (Nov. 22, 2017) 4(4): 86. doi: 10.3390/medicines4040086. pubmed.ncbi.nlm.nih.gov/29165401/?from_term=bacopa+monnieri+and+attention&from_pos=3.

Kean J D, Downey L A, Stough C: A systematic review of the Ayurvedic medicinal herb *Bacopa monnieri* in child and adolescent populations. *Complementary Therapies in Medicine* (Dec. 2016) (29): 56–62. doi: 10.1016/j.ctim.2016.09.002.Epub 2016 Sep 4. pubmed.ncbi.nlm.nih.gov/27912958/?from_term=bacopa+monnieri+and+attention&from_pos=4.

Kellman Raphael MD: *The Microbiome Breakthrough*. New York: Da Capo Press, Hachette Book Group, 2018.

Kenner Dan, Requena Yves: *Botanical Medicine, A European Professional Perspective*. Brookline, MA: Paradigm Publications, 2001.

Khazdair M R, Boskabady M H, Hosseini M, Rezaee R, Tsatsakis A M: The effects of *Crocus sativus* (saffron) and its constituents on nervous system: A review. *Avicenna Journal of Phytomedicine* (Sept.–Oct. 2015) 5(5): 376–391. www.ncbi.nlm.nih.gov/pmc/articles/PMC4599112.

Kim L S, Axelrod L J, Howard P, Buratovich N, Waters R F: Efficacy of methylsulfonylmethane (MSM) in osteoarthritis pain of the knee: A pilot clinical trial. PMID: 16309928 DOI: 10.1016/j.joca.2005.10.003.

Kim Y, et al., Jacobs ET, et al. Vitamin D improves breast cancer survival. *British Journal of Cancer* (2014) 110(11): 2772–2784; *Journal of Cancer* (2016) 7(3): 232–240.

Kuber B R, Thaakur S: Herbs containing L-dopa: An update. *Ancient Science of Life* (Jul., Aug., Sept. 2007) 27(I). www.ncbi.nlm.nih.gov/pmc/articles/PMC3330839/pdf/ASL-27-50.pdf

Linta C: Linking genetics to epigenetics: The role of folate and folate-related pathways in neurodevelopmental disorder. *Clinical Genetics*. First published: 25 July 2018. doi.org/10.1111/ege.13421

Lloyd Brothers*: Cactus grandifloras*. Cincinnati, OH: Lloyd Brothers Cincinnati, 1908. www.swsbm.com/ManualsOther/Selenicereus-Lloyd.PDF.

Lloyd J L: Damiana (Turnera diffusa), 1904. www.herbrally.com/monographs/damiana.

Low Dog T: Vitamin D receptor acts as a transcription factor which regulates cell differentiation. Lecture series in Foundations of Herbal Medicine.

Lyon M R, Cline J C, Totosy de Zepetnek J, Shan J, Pang P, Benishin C: Effect of the herbal extract combination Panax quinquefolium and Ginkgo biloba on attention-deficit hyperactivity. disorder: A pilot study. *Journal of Psychiatry and Neuroscience* (May 2001) 26(3): 221–228. pubmed.ncbi.nlm.nih.gov/11394191.

Mahone E M, Denckla M B: Attention deficit/hyperactivity disorder: A historical neuropsychological perspective. *Journal of the International Psychiatric Society* (Oct. 2017) 23(9–10): 916–929. www.ncbi.nlm.nih.gov/pmc/articles/PMC5724393.

Mancini E, Beglinger C, Drewe J, Zanchi D, Lang U E, Borgwardt S: Green tea effects on cognition, mood and brain function: A systematic review. *Phytomedicine* (Oct. 2017) 15(34): 26–37. doi: 10.1016/j.phymed.2017.07.008.Epub 2017 Jul 27. pubmed.ncbi.nlm.nih.gov/28899506/?from_term=green+tea+for+attention&from_pos=1.

Mansfield K E, Sim J, Jordan J L, Jordan K P: A systematic review and meta-analysis of the prevalence of chronic widespread pain in the general population. *Pain* (Jan. 2016) 157(1). www.ncbi.nlm.nih.gov/pmc/articles/PMC4711387/pdf/jop-157-055.pdf.

Mao J J, Xie S X, Zee J, Soeller I, Li Q S, Rockwell K, Amsterdam J D: *Rhodiola rosea* versus sertraline for major depressive disorder: A randomized placebo-controlled trial. *Phytomedicine* (Mar. 15, 2015) 1(3): 394–399. doi: 10.1016/j.phymed.2015.01.010.Epub 2015 Feb 23. www.ncbi.nlm.nih. gov/pubmed/25837277.

Mayer E A: Bidirection of gut-brain influence on mood etc. Gut feelings: The emerging biology of gut-brain communication. *Nature Reviews Neuroscience* 12(8). doi:10.1038/nrn3071

Mayoclinic.com: Cognitive Behavioral Therapy. www.mayoclinic.org/ tests-procedures/cognitive-behavioral-therapy/about/pac-20384610.

Mendelson, Scott D, MD, PHD: *Herbal Treatment of Major Depression, Scientific Basis and Practical Use.* Boca Raton, FL: CRC Press Taylor and Francis Group, 2020.

Mercola J, Egan B: The Importance of Muscle in Healthy Aging. articles. mercola.com/sites/articles/archive/2020/03/14/skeletal-muscle-aging. aspx.

Mills, S and Bone, K: *Principles and Practice of Phytotherapy Modern Herbal Medicine.* London: Churchill Livingstone, an imprint of Harcourt Publishers Limited, 2000.

Muir S, Montero-Odasso M: Effect of vitamin D supplementation on muscle strength, gait and balance in older adults: A systematic review and meta-analysis. *Journal of the American Geriatric Society* (2011) 59(12): 2291–2300.

Muskin P R: *Complementary and Alternative Medicine and Psychiatry, Review of Psychiatry.* Volume 19. American Psychiatric Press, Inc.

Nathan, Neil, MD: *Toxic: Heal Your Body from Mold Toxicity, Lyme Disease, Multiple Chemical Sensitivities and Chronic Environmental Illness.* Las Vegas, NV: Victory Belt Publishing, 2018.

Neuman H, Debelius J W, Knight R, Koren O. Microbial endocrinology: The interplay between the microbiota and the endocrine system. *FEMS Microbiol Review* (Jul. 2015) 39(4): 509–521. doi: 10.1093/femsre/fuu010.

Neurobehavioral Working Group; Warden D, et al. *Journal of Neurotrauma* (Oct. 2006) 23(10): 1468–1501. pubmed.ncbi.nlm.nih.gov/17020483.

Niederhofer H: Ginkgo biloba treating patients with attention deficit disorder. *Phytotherapy Research* (Jan. 2010) 24(1): 26–27. doi: 10.1002/ptr.2854. pubmed.ncbi.nlm.nih. gov/19441138/?from_term=gingko+biloba+for+add&from_pos=6.

Oubré A: EEG Neurofeedback for treating psychiatric disorders. *Psychiatric Times* (Feb 1, 2002) (19)2. www.psychiatrictimes.com/adhd/ eeg-neurofeedback-treating-psychiatric-disorders/page/0/2.

Park J G, Yi Y-S, Hong Y H, Yoo S, Han S Y, Kim E, Jeong S-G, Aravinthan A, Baik K S, Choi S Y, Son Y-J, Kim J-H: Tabetri™ (*Tabebuia avellandae* ethanol extract) ameliorates osteoarthritis symptoms induced by monoiodoacetate through its anti-inflammatory and chondroprotective activities. *Mediators of Inflammation* (2017): 3619879. Published online

2017 Nov 26. doi: 10.1155/2017/3619879 PMCID: PMC5727801 PMID: 29317792.

Penckofer S, et al.: Vitamin D and depression: Where is all the sunshine? *Issues in Mental Health Nursing* (Jun. 2010) 31(6): 385–393. www.ncbi.nlm.nih.gov/pmc/articles/PMC2908269.

Raškovic A, Milanovic I, Pavlovic N, Cebovic T, Vukmirovic S, Mikov M: Antioxidant activity of rosemary (*Rosmarinus officinalis* L.) essential oil and its hepatoprotective potential. *BMC Complementary and Alternative Medicine* (2014) 14(225). bmccomplementmedtherapies.biomedcentral.com/articles/10.1186/1472-6882-14-225.

Rowland T A, Marwaha S: Epidemiology and risk factors for bipolar disorder. *Therapeautic Advances in Psychopharmacology* (Sept. 2018) 8(9): 251–269. Published online 2018 Apr 26. doi: 10.1177/2045125318769235. PMCID: PMC6116765. PMID: 30181867. www.ncbi.nlm.nih.gov/pmc/articles/PMC6116765/

Sakurai M, et al.: Serum Metabolic Profiles of the tryptophan-kynurenine pathway in the high risk subject of major depressive disorder. *Scientific Reports* (Feb. 6, 2020) 10(1): 1961. doi: 10.1038/s41598-020-58806-w. pubmed.ncbi.nlm.nih.gov/32029791.

Sarkar A, Lehto S M, Harty S, Dinan T G, Cryan J F, Burnet P W J: Psychobiotics and the manipulation of bacteria-gut-brain signals. *Trends in Neuroscience* (Nov. 2016) 39(11): 763–781.

Schöttker B, et al.: Vitamin D and mortality: Meta-analysis of individual participant data from a large consortium of cohort studies from Europe and the United States. *BMJ* (2014) 348: g3656.

Sepalika.com: Gymnema Sylvestre: The Wonder Drug Against Diabetes, December 1, 2016. www.sepalika.com/type-2-diabetes/gymnema-sylvestre-diabetes.

Shannon, Scott M MD: *Mental Health for the Whole Child.* New York: W. W. Norton & Company, 2013.

Shekim W O, Antun F, Hanna G L, McCracken J T, Hess E B: S-Adenosylmethionine (SAM) in Adults with ADHA, RS: Preliminary Results from an Open Trial. *Psychopharmacology bulletin* (1990) 26(2): 249–253. pubmed.ncbi.nlm.nih.gov/2236465.

Shevtsov V A, Zholos B I, Shervarly V I, Volskij V B, Korovin Y P, Khristich M P, Roslyakova NA, Wikman G: A randomized trial of two different doses of a SHR-5 *Rhodiola rosea* extract versus placebo and control of capacity for mental work. *Phytomedicine* (2003) 10(2–3): 95–105. www.sciencedirect.com/science/article/abs/pii/S0944711304702007.

Siblerud R L: The relationship between mercury from dental amalgam and mental health. *American Journal of Psychotherapy* (Apr. 30, 2018). doi.org/10.1176/appi.psychotherapy.1989.43.4.575.

Singh J A, Noorbaloochi S, MacDonald R, Maxwell L J: Chondroitin for osteoarthritis. *Cochrane Database System Review* (Jan. 28, 2015) (1): CD

005614. doi: 10.1002/14651858.CD005614.pub2. pubmed.ncbi.nlm.nih. gov/25629804.

Spinella, Marcello: *The Psychopharmacology of Herbal Medicine, Plant Drugs That Alter Mind, Brain, and Behavior*. Massachusetts Institute of Technology, Cambridge, Massachusetts and London, England, 2001.

Stahl, S M: *Stahl's Essential Psychopharmacology*. Third Edition. New York: Cambridge University Press, 2008.

Stansbury, Jill ND: *Herbal Formularies for Health Professionals. Volume 1. Digestion and Elimination, Including the Gastrointestinal System, Liver and Gall Bladder, Urinary System and the Skin*. White River Junction, VT; London UK: Chelsea Green Publishing, 2018.

Stansbury, Jill ND: *Herbal Formularies for Health Professionals. Volume 4. Neurology, Psychiatry, and Pain Management, Including Cognitive and Neurologic Conditions and Emotional Conditions*. White River Junction, VT; London UK: Chelsea Green Publishing, 2020.

Strickland J, Smith M: The anxiolytic effects of resistance exercise. *Frontiers in Psychology* (2014) (5): 753. www.ncbi.nlm.nih.gov/pmc/articles/ PMC4090891.

Sudarsanan S, Chaudhary S, Pawar A A, Srivastava K: Psychiatric effects of traumatic brain injury. *Medical Journal Armed Forces India* (Jul. 2007) 63(3): 259–263. pubmed.ncbi.nlm.nih.gov/27408012.

Sudo, N: Relationship between the gut microbiome and the hormonal system; the HPAG axis: Microbiome, HPA axis and production of endocrine hormones in the gut. *Advances in Experimental Medicine and Biology* (2014) (817): 177–194. 10.1007/978-1-4939-0897-4_8.

Talbott S, Talbott J, Pugh M: Effect of *Magnolia officinalis* and *Phellodendron amurense* (Relora®) on cortisol and psychological mood state in moderately stressed subjects. *Journal of the International Society of Sports Nutrition* (2013) 10(37): 9. jissn.biomedcentral.com/articles/10.1186/1550-2783-10-37.

Thompson K: Ashwagandha (*Withania somnifera*). www.herbrally.com/ monographs/ashwagandha.

ThyroidAdvisor.com: *Bacopa monnieri*—Effects and benefits on the Thyroid Gland. April 4, 2017.

Tilgner, Sharol Marie ND: *Herbal Medicine from the Heart of the Earth, Expanded Materia Medica and Formulas*. Third Edition. Pleasant Hill, OR: Wise Acres, 2020.

Trebatická J, Kopasová S, Hradecná Z, Cinovský K, Skodáček I, Suba J, Muchova J, Zitnanová I, Waczulíková I, Rohdewald P, Durackova Z: Treatment of ADHD with French maritime bark extract, Pycnogenol®. Randomized controlled trial. *European Child & Adolescent Psychiatry* (Sept. 2006) 15(6): 329–335. pubmed.ncbi.nlm.nih.gov/16699814.

Tremellen K et al.: Metabolic endotoxaemia—a potential novel link between ovarian inflammation and impaired progesterone production. *Gynecological Endocrinology* (Apr. 2015) 31(4): 309–312. doi: 10.3109/09513590.2014.994602.

van Calker D, Bibert K, Domschke K, Serchov T: The role of adenosine receptors in mood and anxiety disorders. *Journal of Neurochemistry* (2019) (151): 11–27. onlinelibrary.wiley.com/doi/pdf/10.1111/jnc.14841.

Vasquez, Alex, DC ND: *Musculoskeletal Pain: Expanded Clinical Strategies*. Gig Harbor, WA: The Institute for Functional Medicine, 2008.

Walsh, WJ: *Nutrient Power, Heal Your Biochemistry and Heal Your Brain*. New York: Skyhorse Publishing, 2004.

Wang C, Gao H, Cai E, Zhang L, Zheng X, Zhang S, Sun N, Zhao Y: Protective effects of *Acanthopanax senticosus-Ligustrum lucidum* combination on bone marrow suppression induced chemotherapy in mice. *Biomedicine & Pharmacotherapy* (Jan. 2019) (109): 2062–2069. doi: 10.1016/j. biopha.2018.11.071.Epub 2018 Nov 26. www.ncbi.nlm.nih.gov/ pubmed/30551462

Wang X, Li P, Pan C, Dai L, Wu Y, Deng Y: The Effect of Mind-Body Therapies on Insomnia: A Systematic Review and Meta-analysis. Evidence based complementary and Alternative Medicine. 2019 Article ID 9359807. doi.org/10.1155/2019/9359807. www.hindawi.com/ journals/ecam/2019/9359807.

Webmd: Saffron: www.webmd.com/vitamins/ai/ingredientmono-844/saffron

Weinstein J: Quick study Craft cooking Chef's Guide Herbs and Spices, 2018 BarCharts Publishing, In. 1118

Weinstein S J et al.: Vitamin D and colon cancer survival: Lower mortality every 10 ng/ml your D goes up it confers 29% improvement of mortality. *International Journal of Cancer* (2014). doi:10.1002/ijc.29157.

Whitaker, Robert: *Anatomy of an Epidemic*. New York: Broadway Paperbacks, 2010.

Winston, D RH(AHG), with Steven L. Maimes: *Adaptogens, Herbs for Strength, Stamina, and Stress Relief*. Rochester, VT: Healing Arts Press, 2019.

Winston, David RH(AHG): *Herbal Therapeutics*. Broadway, NJ: Herbal Therapeutics Research Library, 2019.

Xiao H, Tan C, Yang G, Dou D: The effect of red ginseng and ginseng leaves on the substance and energy metabolism in hypothyroidism rats. (Oct. 2017) 41(4): 556–565. doi: 10.1016/j. jgr.2016.11.005. Epub 2017 Jan 16. pubmed.ncbi.nlm.nih. gov/29021704/?from_term=red+ginseng+and+thyroid&from_pos=1.

Zhu X, Sang L, Wu D, Rong J, Jiang L: Effectiveness and safety of glucosamine and chondroitin for the treatment of osteoarthritis: A meta-analysis of randomized controlled trials. Journal of Orthopaedic Surgery and Research (2018) (13): 170. Published online 2018 Jul 6. doi: 10.1186/ s13018-018-0871-5. PMCID: PMC6035477 PMID: 29980200.

ACKNOWLEDGMENTS

I would like to thank Maureen O'Malley for her tireless review of my work to keep it simple.

I would like to thank my husband, Stanley Armstrong, for being my biggest fan.

I would like to thank Dr. Daniel Amen for encouraging all those who work for him to reach out on their own.

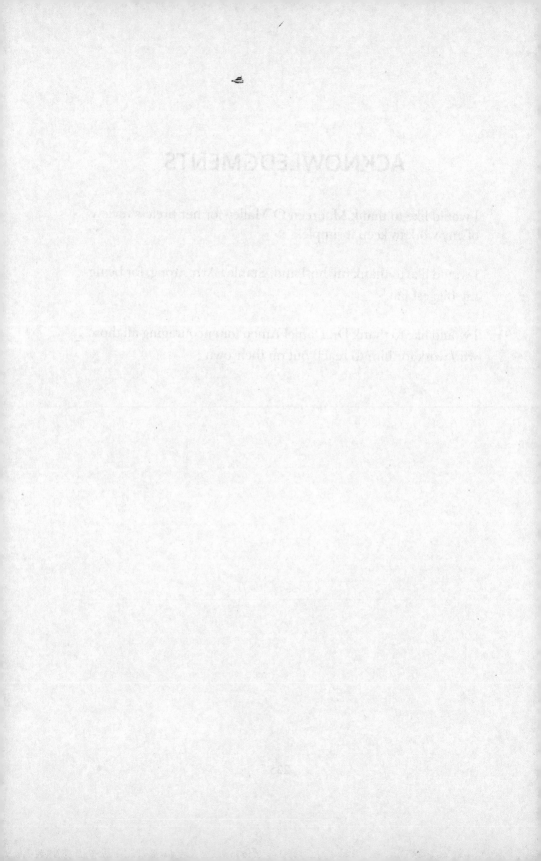

INDEX

Visit us online at
KensingtonBooks.com
to read more from your favorite authors,
see books by series, view reading
group guides, and more!

BOOK   CLUB
BETWEEN THE CHAPTERS

Visit us online for sneak peeks, exclusive
giveaways, special discounts, author content,
and engaging discussions with your fellow readers.

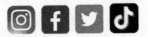
Betweenthechapters.net

Sign up for our newsletters and be the first
to get exciting news and announcements about
your favorite authors!
Kensingtonbooks.com/newsletter